INNER
SECRETS

INNER SECRETS

Discovering T'ai Chi's Hidden
Lessons *for* Preservation,
Protection, *and* Peace of Mind

WILLIAM DONNELLY

ISBN: 9798987955901 (print)
ISBN: 9798987955918 (epub)

Cover and Interior Book Design: Happenstance Type-O-Rama

Published by
Apeirogon Publishing
Patchogue, New York

For Regina, a feather in the wind

Ancient art has a specific inner content. At one time art possessed the same purpose that books do in our day, namely: to perceive and transmit knowledge. In olden days, people did not write books, they incorporated their knowledge into works of art. We would find a great many ideas in the works of ancient art passed down to us, if we only knew how to read them.

—GEORGE GURDJIEFF

CONTENTS

FOREWORD

*An Excellent Guide
to T'ai Chi*

T'ai Chi (*Taiji*, or "grand ultimate") Chuan (*Quan*, or "fist") is an ancient Chinese art. Some people might conjure up an image of an old Chinese man dressed in loose white silk pajamas, slowly and gracefully moving his arms and legs in a park early in the morning, before the fog has dispersed. Some recognize that T'ai Chi is great for health but think they're not old enough for it, assuming that T'ai Chi is good only for seniors who are too old to do any other type of exercise. Actually, T'ai Chi is good not just for seniors but for anyone and everyone.

A multitude of scientific studies in recent decades conducted by prominent Western medical research institutes have proven that T'ai Chi provides extensive health benefits, including but not limited to easing or eliminating chronic pains; regaining physical balance; reducing stress, anxiety, and depression; enhancing cardiovascular functions; delaying the onset of dementia; improving sleep quality; enriching overall life quality; and speeding up cancer recovery.

Many doctors now advise their patients to take up T'ai Chi to improve various health conditions. Veterans Affairs physicians are now prescribing T'ai Chi instead of pills as a medical intervention for several diseases. Millions are now trying T'ai Chi as a healing art.

Once, in one of my T'ai Chi classes, I mentioned that T'ai Chi is not just a healing art but also a martial art. Instantly, a few ladies' eyes popped wider; these women were probably wondering whether they were attending the wrong class. On the contrary, several gentlemen grinned with excitement. Male students who used to practice hard-style martial arts like Karate or Taekwondo switched to T'ai Chi because it's easier on their aging bodies, suggesting that T'ai Chi Chuan is an old man's martial art. That's somewhat true, but not entirely.

In China, the state-run TV broadcaster China Central Television has hosted martial arts tournaments, most of which are organized by styles or categories—for example, Wing Chun versus Wing Chun, and Shaolin versus Shaolin. Occasionally, they host a grand championship where the winners of different styles/categories fight against each other to determine who is the grand champion among all of the martial arts styles. T'ai Chi Chuan has overcome the others a few times. T'ai Chi champions even take down the champions of Japanese Sumo wrestling and Thai Muay Thai.

Historically, T'ai Chi is considered the grand martial art in China, even though it appears to be very slow and gentle. It's extremely powerful and especially advantageous for people who are small in stature and don't have bulging muscles, because T'ai Chi Chuan teaches practitioners how to borrow the incoming brute force and deflect it. Thus, it's excellent for women to learn for the purpose of self-defense.

I was invited by a library to teach T'ai Chi as a health awareness program to a group who had never experienced it. My topic was the Silk Reeling or Spiraling, which is a seemingly simple yet nuanced regimen. First, I demonstrated it. Right before I was going to instruct how to do it, a lady raised her hand and stated that the Silk Reeling looked easy enough, and that she could close her eyes and imagine she was practicing on a mountain-top and feeling the spirit. Yes, this century-old exercise is perceived by some as a New Age spiritual ritual.

To many long-term practitioners, T'ai Chi is an enlightenment (though not a religion). It is a way of thinking and an attitude toward life, nature, relationships, and values—essentially a *way of life*. T'ai Chi Chuan itself does not actually teach us these perspectives. However, through studying and practicing the T'ai Chi Chuan fundamentals established for the body movements, people gradually comprehend the profundity of the underlying philosophy. Some grasp this wisdom quickly, and others discover it more slowly.

It doesn't matter how soon you find out about the many facets of the art, because T'ai Chi is what you make of it, and it is very personal. However, the brilliance of *Inner Secrets*, written by Sifu Bill Donnelly, can shed some light on your T'ai Chi journey regardless of whether you are learning the physical exercise or just want to have a better and more holistic comprehension of it.

As a T'ai Chi examiner for over a decade with a global readership of forty-plus countries, I feel the responsibility to bring every aspect of the art to readers. I have written more than seven hundred articles, mostly in English and some in Chinese. The majority of my writings are published online. I have the privilege of interviewing top-notch scientists around the world to discuss the health benefits of this healing art. I interview masters, grandmasters, and experts regarding the practice's philosophy, principles, theories, and techniques. I also speak with practitioners of all walks of life to understand how the art affects them physically, emotionally, and spiritually.

Sifu Bill Donnelly is a lineage holder of Choy Li Fut (a Chinese martial art) and a longtime Yang-style T'ai Chi practitioner. He has also taught T'ai Chi for over twenty years. He has a successful career recruiting and coaching executives in the financial industry. Additionally, he is an established musician and plays drums with groups for recordings and live shows at various venues in New York City. Impressed by his versatile talents, I interviewed Bill and wrote a story about him a few years ago. Later, I realized that Bill has a passion for writing as well. At my request, he wrote a couple of articles for my online publication *VioletLiTaiChi.com* and received excellent feedback from readers.

In March 2020, the country started to shut down due to the COVID-19 pandemic. To help people fight against the virus and improve their immune systems, I founded a Free T'ai Chi and Qigong lesson program and live-streamed it to 30 countries, getting over 400,000 total views for approximately 150 episodes. Bill was a generous soul and took time out of his busy schedule to appear as a guest instructor. He is extremely methodical. His lessons were hard and required much concentration and stamina, but the payback was rewarding and helped students deepen their knowledge and skill.

Besides being experienced in T'ai Chi theory and practice, Bill is well read and articulate. In *Inner Secrets*, he explains T'ai Chi from several aspects so readers can have a 360-degree view. He employs real-life stories to expound why T'ai Chi matters and how its principles can be applied to solve problems, conflicts, and dilemmas in daily life.

If you are practicing T'ai Chi Chuan, *Inner Secrets* can help you understand why and how to adhere to the T'ai Chi fundamentals to elevate your skills. Even if you haven't tried T'ai Chi Chuan and have no intention of learning, Bill's book provides a clear vision with a refreshing approach to more easily manage relationships with family, friends, coworkers, and even strangers. *Inner Secrets* can also assist you in navigating your career path or business plan, especially in an era when uncertainty is the only sure thing.

Even though Bill asserts that *Inner Secrets* is not a how-to book, it does reveal the secrets of the art of T'ai

Chi Chuan. Discover his silent flow of wisdom through this easy read, which provides a road map for a more fulfilling life for all readers.

—VIOLET LI, founder of "Tai Chi and
Qigong for Health" and *VioletLiTaiChi.com*

GENERAL HISTORICAL TIMELINE OF T'AI CHI

Dates and credits are approximate, do not include the many interim contributors, and are presented here as a historical timeline of development.

1122 BC	Yi Jing's *The I Ching*, or *The Book of Changes*, introduces the concept of Yin and Yang.
502 AD	Basic principles of T'ai Chi Chuan emerge, taught by Han Gong-Yue.
600 AD	Philosopher Lao Tzu connects the Yin and Yang to man and nature; establishes Taoism.
618 AD	Thirty-Seven Postures, with martial techniques, are taught with similar T'ai Chi Chuan concepts.
1101 AD	Zhang San-Feng, a Wudang Taoist, is the recognized creator of T'ai Chi Chuan techniques. The common origin story depicts Zhang San-Feng observing a fight between a crane and a snake, thus inspiring a natural approach to the martial art.
1100–1500 AD	T'ai Chi developed and transmitted through individuals, eventually dividing into northern and southern styles.

1540 AD	The Chen family establishes Old-Style and New-Style T'ai Chi, which is preserved through exclusive family transmission.
1799 AD	Yang Lu-Chan is born. Yang, an outsider, learns and masters the Chen family T'ai Chi style and incorporates Taoist yoga, thus softening the overall style and creating the Yang-style branch of T'ai Chi.
1834 AD	Wu Quan-Yu is born. He trains in Yang-style T'ai Chi and later develops Wu-style T'ai Chi.
1833 AD	Li I-yu is born. He studies Wu T'ai Chi and develops the Li branch of T'ai Chi.
1861 AD	Sun Lu-Tang, an accomplished martial artist, trains in Wu/Hao T'ai Chi at fifty years old. He incorporates concepts that characterize Sun T'ai Chi.
1960s AD	Cheng Man Ch'ing arrives in New York and brings T'ai Chi to America.
21st century	Western medical institutions, including Harvard Medical School, publish studies on the benefits of T'ai Chi.

NOTE TO READER

Make Your Own Mantra

Reading a book is just the beginning of learning a new idea or concept. The next important step is to integrate this new knowledge in a way that becomes a part of us. One way to solidify a takeaway from this book is to make your own mantra.

I regularly annotate the books I read. Several years ago I realized what the next step could be. I began to review the highlighted areas to extract the essential words, then restructure them into a more concise phrase that is easier to remember. To illustrate the process, I'll use the following passage, which was edited out of the final draft of this book. If I highlighted this passage as a reader, then my process would be:

STEP 1: SELECT YOUR ESSENTIAL WORDS FROM HIGHLIGHTED PASSAGE.

All things that exist in **nature** have a **symmetry**. **Water**, for instance, naturally seeks a state of balance when it fills a void, rolls down a river, or crashes in waves.

When rapidly careening down a mountainside, water will alter its path to dissipate the energy.

Water nourishes plants, animals, and humans. It offers **benefits without thought or emotion and without seeking gratitude, recognition, or compensation**. It simply **Flows**.

Since we as people are composed of about 60 percent water, we can flow, too. We can seek balance and change our path to disperse constant rushing energy, which may be stress, anger, frustration, etc. When we flow like water, we are **expressing the highest state of our nature**.

STEP 2: ASSEMBLE THE HIGHLIGHTED KEY WORDS.

Nature; symmetry; water; benefits without thought or emotion and without seeking gratitude, recognition, or compensation; flows; expressing the highest state of our nature.

STEP 3: BE CREATIVE WITH THE ORDER UNTIL YOU FIND A PHRASE THAT PERSONALLY RESONATES.

I flow like water,
Offering benefit without thought or emotion,
Not seeking gratitude, recognition, or compensation
My highest state of nature exists.

This process reminds me of Buddhist chants I learned. I shared this with a Buddhist monk, who said it was a right path. Making your own mantra is fun, creative, and highly personal, so you will be inspired to repeat it often—because it is *yours*. The repetition is what creates lasting change and mastery. Go through the book, find your notes or favorite passages, then make them your own. Experiment and enjoy.

INTRODUCTION

Every decision, action, and emotion has an origin or cause. It can be generated from an occurrence that had some impact on you, even if only minimal. My gravitation to T'ai Chi was a result of understanding and developing newly discovered strengths. But that experience occurs later. Before that, this origin story of my entry into martial arts, specifically kung fu, was a response to a life-changing event.

I arrived home from work in the dark, as the late fall season shortened the days. My wife, Jeanne, greeted me as usual, but her gestures were short, a courteous formality that moved past our normal routine and on to something that was on her mind. She walked to the phone and began to dial a number.

"I want you to listen to something," she said.

I waited while my wife connected into her work phone system and extension. She entered the passcode and put on the speakerphone. The voice of a man, low in tone to control anger or rage, spoke one sentence we will never forget: "If I see you again, I will kill you, bitch."

Jeanne surveyed my face for a reaction. When she played the message to her manager and the owner of the company, they dismissed the call and walked away. Jeanne wanted to see if I concurred.

I did not.

We called the police, who promptly arrived and listened to the message. The officer's response was as serious as ours. The officer was ready to act.

The police officer asked my wife if she knew who the caller was. Jeanne immediately thought of a problematic employee whom she was never comfortable around. This person was recently terminated and may have identified Jeanne as the cause, or a target for retaliation. Without being 100 percent sure, and unwilling to falsely accuse someone, Jeanne would not commit to identifying this person as the perpetrator.

The next day I decided to establish a presence and demonstrate protection by driving her to work. As I left her and started the drive to my office, an uncomfortable feeling began to creep up, as if I'd just delivered a lamb to the slaughter. Now my wife was in a building with lax, unaware, and self-centered management, and without a car or another means to escape. If something were to occur, what could I do when my office was an hour-long drive away?

I decided to take the day off to stay close to home, clear my head, and think through what to do in response. I began to write anything that came to mind—pages of assessments, concerns, fears, options, fantasies, and questions, like:

- I could give her pepper spray. But in real terms, this would likely wind up at the bottom of her handbag.

- A gun or knife wasn't a better option, because unless she was committed to using the weapon it could be easily taken and used against her.

- What could I give her that could not be taken away?

The answer that came to me: *knowledge.*

If I could help my wife gain knowledge of how to protect herself, then she would have a greater advantage and an increased potential to survive in any situation. Knowledge is indeed real power. I just had to find that knowledge.

I stopped in to visit a nearby kung fu school that had recently opened. I anticipated a ten-minute conversation but sat with Sifu (Master Instructor) Gus Kaparos, the owner, for over half an hour as he listened, offered information, and answered my questions. I left the meeting thinking that this man must be an accomplished martial artist, because not once did he mention how good he was.

I proposed to Jeanne that we try a few classes, and if she was comfortable, we would begin to train. For the next few years, we attended classes together. Jeanne's confidence grew, and accordingly, conflicts and challengers began to disappear. Her life began to change.

I went all in. I trained in kung fu, and was eventually ranked a black belt and accepted into the Choy Li Fut lineage. While doing that, and less than a year into my training, I decided to take a T'ai Chi class. Then *my* life began to change.

* * *

This work is an expression of the knowledge I have gained through the study of T'ai Chi. It is a result of studying and practicing to master the form and understand its health and self-defense applications, but more broadly to understand why and how this art can be used in one's life. Over the last twenty years I have read the T'ai Chi classics, along with the *Tao de Ching* and *The Art of War*, and have spoken with and observed peers, colleagues, and martial arts Sifus. And finally, I have reflected on my own experience during the ups and downs of daily living.

The book is about T'ai Chi, but more than that it's about everything I've learned about life through the practice of this art. I couldn't do better at delivering details of the form and its application than the many authors before me, who possess more experience and higher skills than I do. And what would be the point? The world doesn't need another "how to" book. What I offer here is not *how* we should practice an art like T'ai Chi, but rather *why*. Why should someone consider this path—a longer and more demanding path than most—over other forms of exercise or self-defense? What can be divined from a daily practice of T'ai Chi that could enhance one's life beyond good health? Here I set out to raise awareness of what I've gleaned from this multifaceted art. It has demanded patience, but my effort has been rewarded.

Any book will reflect a truth, but it is a truth discovered by the book's author. That is what *Inner Secrets* is. My intent is to raise your awareness through my experiences so that you may discover your own truth in life. If, through my observation and reporting, you can draw a personal parallel or make your own discovery, thus bringing you closer to your personal truth, then I have succeeded.

I am offering answers to the questions most asked of me, including: Why is T'ai Chi so slow? Is it really a workout? Is it really a form of self-defense? How can T'ai Chi improve my life? Where else can these concepts and precepts be used? Some of the answers I found are wide-ranging. Some points may seem unrelated but ultimately lead to the common theme, just from a different angle, like facets of a diamond. That's because one element of learning T'ai Chi will naturally enhance another. For instance, when we focus on the physical attributes of T'ai Chi, it influences our health. Health will impact our frame of mind. Health and the right frame of mind raise the spirit. You'll find some passages may require more than a casual read, but with a little time and attention they can open a new way of thinking.

The essays are arranged in a sequence but can be read in any order you like. And you don't need to read this book in one sitting. For the person seeking greater understanding and fulfillment in their T'ai Chi practice, this book may be an ideal companion. The intention is to open a door of awareness along your path to discover self-knowledge.

WHAT IS T'AI CHI?

*A Basic Introduction to the
Core Components of T'ai Chi*

P erhaps T'ai Chi appears strange and mysterious to a person from the Western Hemisphere because the point of origin is different than their own experiences. If we were to compare religions like Christianity to Buddhism, for instance, we might broadly characterize one as perceiving that the great mystery exists outside of us, while the other believes the mystery is within ourselves. From the vantage point of a Westerner—more or less raised and influenced by a European history, philosophy, culture, and religion—an art like T'ai Chi, when viewed in isolation, may seem strange, foreign, or just plain weird. Or even worse: New Age.

Over the last five decades, many Westerners have been exposed to the contributions of the Far East through circumstance or curiosity—for example, by serving as soldiers, marrying Chinese immigrants, or doing their own research as artists and flower children. As a result,

T'ai Chi, kung fu, and yoga have permeated the Western subconscious. Yoga has become the most popular, but I believe that its acceptance is based more on the challenge of the physical exercise than the psychological benefits of the practice. If that's the case, then an art like T'ai Chi, which offers multiple benefits, has a long way to go in terms of educating the Western masses.

To the uninitiated, Taosim, the underlying philosophy of T'ai Chi, conjures images of a mystical sage. In fact, with study and increased awareness of the intention, purpose, and lessons contained within the poetic writing of the *Tao de Ching*, you begin to understand that it's not as esoteric as you might have originally believed.

To understand T'ai Chi, we must understand its components. T'ai Chi represents the culmination of three uniquely integrated disciplines: Qi Gong, including meditation; the philosophy of Taoism; and martial arts as self-defense. These three elements developed independently and eventually merged over hundreds of years. This is what makes T'ai Chi singular and rich. The history, depth, and subtlety contained within each element of T'ai Chi invite a lifetime of practice, exploration, and learning. So, let's begin at the beginning: What is Qi?

Everyone is born with a certain level of inherent energy, or what the Chinese call *Qi* (pronounced "chee"). Energy is created when the body processes food and air. The quality of each impacts the quality of Qi energy.

Qi exists in each part of the body, including blood cells and organs. Each will function best with an optimum level of Qi. Too little, and the organ doesn't function properly. Too much, and the organ may burn out or degenerate more rapidly.

Qi Gong is the study and development of Qi (energy) through Gong (effort or work to achieve mastery). Qi Gong theory divides the mind into two parts: the wisdom mind and the emotional mind. The wisdom mind brings an idea into action as a physical event. The emotional mind is where you feel upset, tension, anger, and the like. By learning to use the wisdom mind to control the emotional mind, you become better at addressing life's challenges and contributing to society. This transformation is achieved with meditation, which is the root of Qi Gong and T'ai Chi.

Meditation mediates the inner conflict that resides within our nature. The root principle is balancing our emotions, not reaching the extremes. This is a practice of harmonizing love and loathing, giving and taking, violence and nonviolence. Like religious prayer, meditation is used to gain peace of mind. If you've ever sat quietly watching a campfire or relaxed at the beach watching endless waves crest and fall, then you've unknowingly slipped into a state of meditation.

T'ai Chi, and the underlying Taoist philosophy, is a system of thought and does not require devotion to a God, deity, or object in order to create peace of mind. The body, mind, and spirit interconnect through Qi to create a total living, healthy being. Qi is moved by concentrating the mind, which improves the energy of the physical body. The mind and body's energetic interaction creates a resonance, which raises the spirit.

According to the historical timeline, early scholarly and religious practitioners in the East believed that spiritual life was more important than physical life, so they tended toward still or sitting meditation. This group also believed that an emotionally balanced mind was the key component of good health.

Over time the work of China's medical doctors, who discovered Qi approximately four thousand years ago, began to gain acceptance, and physical development became recognized as a critical component to good health. The doctors integrated Qi Gong exercises—still rooted in meditation—into their acupuncture and herbal practices. Many of these theories and practices were developed before 206 BC, the year of the earliest recording of the Qi Gong systems. In this system, physical development evolved out of mindfulness. This is a unique attribute of T'ai Chi.

The Science of Qi Gong

The Qi circulating in our bodies is essentially bioelectricity that exists as an electromagnetic field. This energy can be positively or negatively influenced by the good or bad energy that surrounds us, including weather patterns, our mood, and the emotional energy of people around us. The stronger your Qi, the less likely you are to experience mood swings or illness, and the slower your aging process.

Qi Gong is a natural science that studies energy in all forms, including energy found in the human body, the earth, the atmosphere, and our universe. The purpose of Qi Gong training is to conserve the body's energy and improve its quality. Qi Gong training sustains the movement of energy smoothly and without obstruction.

Qi Gong is also a great way to eliminate toxins. T'ai Chi, which is considered a facet of Qi Gong, includes movements based on spirals, which are found everywhere in nature. Our galaxy is a spiral, as are the orbit of the planets, the spinning of the Earth, the flow of water down a drain, and the beginning of a storm or a tornado. By using this spiral movement in the T'ai Chi techniques, a person is twisting muscles and applying pressure to parts of the body. Twisting limits the flow of blood into the area and untwisting releases it in a rush, cleaning out the organ, artery, or vein. The spiraling pattern is also used to generate power in martial applications.

Qi Gong has always treated the body and mind as integrated, not separate parts. This differs from current Western practices, where some people watch TV while doing their exercise. Their body is engaged in one thing, and their mind in another. The mind's shift in focus and intent away from their body and toward distractions creates separation. Why does this matter?

The Mind/Body Connection

Our body and mind are connected by the nervous system, which is made of physical, electrical, and chemical elements. The nervous system begins at the brain and connects to muscles and tendons, allowing the brain to control the actions of the body. The messages sent from the brain to the body, or vice versa, influence our mood, emotions, and physical perceptions of the environment or events around us. Any break in this link is a distraction and can have serious consequences (think texting while driving).

The Philosophy of Taoism

If Qi Gong is the science of nature, then Taoism is best described as the philosophy of nature. Taoism is based on the natural duality that exists within all things and originates from one source. Negative and positive energy, day and night, life and death, up and down, hot and cold, success and failure, male and female, positive and negative charges, full and empty—these are a few of the myriad examples. It is best illustrated in the Yin Yang symbol: the interaction of black and white, each containing a piece of the other.

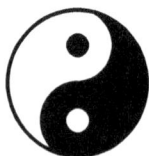

Hence, when someone looks at the world in this way, they're no longer singularly focused, and become less biased in their view. You see the world more clearly and objectively and respond in a more spontaneous and relevant way. The response is in accordance with your personal nature, which increasingly aligns with universal nature through continued study and practice.

Taoism also exists in Western thought and can be found in the writings of contemporary philosophers Henry David Thoreau (1817–1862) and Ralph Waldo Emerson (1803–1882). The Stoic philosophers, including Marcus Aurelius, embraced concepts very similar to Taoism. Aurelius called Qi the creative fire, composed of water, earth, and air. The Chinese would call it the five elements: wood, fire, earth, metal, and water. Modern Western science calls it physics.

Around 502 AD, Qi Gong evolved into martial practice, which is divided into external and internal sides. External martial arts are focused on developing strong musculature for power. Internal martial arts, including T'ai Chi, Xingyi, and Bagua styles, generate power from internal Qi and move it to the limbs, which, when relaxed, allow the energy to flow unobstructed. Sometimes internal styles need muscle, too, but that's not the primary approach.

So, if a person uses Qi for strength, will it work? Is there proof? Some of these attributes present themselves spontaneously.

I watched a news report from Logan, Utah, where an injured motorcyclist was rescued by several pedestrian heroes. The man was traveling eastbound on Route 89 when a BMW pulled out of a parking lot and struck the motorcycle, pinning the cyclist and severing the bike's fuel line. A fire broke out.

Eight people rushed to the car and tried unsuccessfully to lift the four-thousand-pound vehicle. The group thought the man was dead and were trying to recover the body instead of letting it burn. But then one woman decided to lie down on the ground to assess one more time.

Her eyes connected with the biker's and she yelled, "He's still alive!" The group rushed back to the car, successfully lifting it this time, and pulled the man from the wreckage, saving his life.

People rightfully called the group heroes and their feat a miracle. But others have asked how can a group of people, each with enough strength to lift a couple hundred pounds at most, be strong enough to lift this four-thousand-pound vehicle, especially when they couldn't do it only moments earlier?

The answer is that the woman's cry raised the group's spirit, triggering a release of energy that increased each person's muscle strength beyond its normal capacity. Some call it a miracle. The Chinese call it Qi Gong.

All of us have the potential to develop this capacity. Although we may never be called upon to respond to a challenge this great, we face many everyday challenges. We can learn to cultivate Qi for the power to meet those challenges, just as the Chinese discovered in 1108 AD.

T'ai Chi as a Martial Art

The T'ai Chi form (sequence) combines the philosophical, Qi Gong, and martial arts disciplines for health and self-preservation. Encoded in the form are fighting applications, including techniques to bring an opponent down with pushes, throws and takedowns, joint locks, and cavity strikes. Each technique contains an energy pattern that begins from a state of calm and relaxation, then generates a focused surge of power that progresses to an explosive release. These techniques keep the body relaxed and agile, allowing it to move continuously without muscle tension, which blocks or burns energy inefficiently.

T'ai Chi fighting techniques are based on remaining in contact with the opponent to sense their movement or intention, and then neutralizing their attack by yielding and redirecting it. This strategy enables you to lead and control the opponent.

The strategy is not to fight force with force. It is to reduce or eliminate incoming force through "no resistance," getting the opponent to overcommit, which uses their power against them. The opponent's Yang energy becomes Yin. People might recognize this as "fighting by not fighting" or "doing without doing."

If you were one of the millions who watched Super Bowl XLVI between the New England Patriots and the New York Giants, then you likely saw one of T'ai Chi's leading principles in action. Let's review the play-by-play.

It is the fourth quarter at the two-minute warning: Giants, 15; Patriots, 17. The Giants are in the end zone with their fourth down. Their plan is to run the ball to the one-yard line and stay there in order to run down the clock. After that, a touchdown and field goal kick will give the team their points and eliminate any remaining time for a Patriots comeback.

Giants quarterback Eli Manning hands off the ball to Ahmad Bradshaw, who focuses his energy to force through the defenders and get to the one-yard line. Off he goes into the mob. But instead of pushing, tackling, or grabbing, Bradshaw finds something he never anticipated: no resistance. The Patriots simply stepped aside, clearing a path for Bradshaw to charge through. Bradshaw, now overcommitted, cannot stop himself from the touchdown. Even trying to squat at the line, Bradshaw fell on his butt and scored a touchdown, leaving enough time on the clock for one last attempt by the Patriots.

It's rare to see this strategy in a sport like football. It seems counterintuitive. But it worked (although the Patriots ultimately lost the game).

T'ai Chi training develops your focus, using a high level of concentration to direct your Qi energy, or bioelectricity, to specific areas of the body. This increases the efficient transfer of energy and overall power beyond the 40 percent average. The ability to concentrate energy in a specific area increases personal strength substantially. The highly trained people of internal martial arts strike with substantial power and are able to resist blows to the body, thus reducing injury.

The fighting strategy of T'ai Chi can be applied to many areas, including negotiation and conflict resolution. It also can help someone look at the macro picture and become more intuitive and artful in how they solve problems or create opportunities. T'ai Chi helps you practice a mindset that can be applied to the numerous challenges of daily living in a healthy way.

The Way of T'ai Chi in a Modern World

The world is changing every day, but even more significantly now. Life and living in the twenty-first century evolves at a faster pace than any century before. It races the heart and the mind. We must practice a way of thinking that allows the brain to function in a more lucid and mindful manner. T'ai Chi is the practice of awareness, rejuvenation, and creativity that supports the underlying principle of self-renewal.

The dramatic changes our economy and society are currently experiencing will likely persist for several years. Professional and personal survival will require our ability to adapt. The root of adaptation lies in creativity, along with physical, emotional, and mental flexibility; without these tools, people become resistant to change, which often leads to frustration, depression, and illness.

The practice of T'ai Chi is an opportunity to cultivate self-knowledge and self-development for a lifetime. It offers philosophical, health, and relationship-strengthening techniques that can be learned, studied, developed, and applied to daily life. You may choose to practice each day or a few times a week. The more you put into T'ai Chi, the more you'll get out of it.

It's been said that we are what we eat, we are what we wear, we are what we watch, but really, we are what we do. We create patterns and habits that reinforce our mindsets and values. T'ai Chi supports a mindset that is critically needed at this time.

T'ai Chi is a historically proven way to improve your mental and physical well-being in a world driven by the uncertainty of global politics, personal conflict, and environmental, economic, and health-care challenges.

T'ai Chi is a system of survival.

T'ai Chi is a way of life.

THE *TAO DE CHING*

Small Book of Timeless Wisdom

T'ai Chi is the only health system and martial art created with philosophy at its foundation. It is based on the philosophy of Taosim, which is imparted in the *Tao de Ching*, written almost 2,500 years ago. The work is credited to Lao Tzu, a sixth-century BC sage who studied nature in order to comprehend life. The text of the *Tao de Ching* has been interpreted and adapted to instruct on Qi Gong practice, martial strategy, and personal conduct. It is a timeless and treasured document that was birthed from a dark period in China's history.

The *Tao de Ching* was written during China's Warring States period, a brutal era that transitioned from the old order to a new and uncertain state of society and politics. As early as 770 BC, during the Eastern Zhou period, the Shi, who functioned as priests or as knights, emerged; they were educated and existed at a level akin to the modern middle class.

Societal changes bred new and more complex challenges. Rulers struggled to protect their people and borders while promoting welfare. It was from this need that Confucius, Mencius, Sunzi, and other great thinker/philosopher-advisors came to prominence. Drawing on lessons of the past—best practices, as we now call them—they created an overarching perspective from which they could advise the rulers. Although schools of thought differed among the Shi, they commonly believed that a ruler must act in accordance with the principles of the natural universe, possess ethics and morality, and lead by example. Additionally, the Shi believed that the basic nature of people was good. Wrongdoing among the populace was a result of poor structures and leadership.

Since human beings are social creatures that communicate and interact, the Shi realized that an ideal combination of words could influence their behavior. They began to communicate through verse. The words universally applied to circumstance, adversity, conflict, and challenges. These verses became a guiding principle for leadership and self-governance.

It was Confucius that introduced and advocated the self-cultivation of morality to create inner harmony. The concept of inner harmony was developed further in the writings within the text of *Guanzi*, in a section of the document known as Inner Training. This method was created to balance the extremes in mental and emotional states. Emptying oneself through physical exercise aligns the body and the mind by cultivating and directing one's energy, or Qi.

An empty mind heightens our perception of the subtle patterns of behavior that exist in all of nature, including human interaction. We stop labeling and categorizing, which are behaviors based solely on perception. We become more aware of reality: the guiding principles of the universe. By cultivating a sense of the order and flow of nature, we become adept at living in accordance with events as they occur, responding spontaneously according to our own nature.

Periods of savage war, changes in politics (as tribes overthrew each other and changed the system of rule), and new social structures produced profound levels of thought and philosophical systems. The change of consciousness provided a foundation for people to thrive. It was as critical to survival then as it is now.

Many would argue that our society has entered a dark period over the last quarter century. As of this writing, the US continues to be engaged in significant conflict. There is a divided and increasingly rancorous government. Opposing countries are accused of using cyberattacks to influence elections and divide citizens. Our environment is in turmoil, as evidenced by the increase in severe storms, extreme temperatures, droughts, and floods, and wreaking havoc on plants and animals. The world economy has not grown and debt is increasing.

What is widely missing during this time of significant challenges and rapid, sometimes unforgiving change is a culture of self-cultivation based on principles that guide individuals and leaders to make sound decisions and take appropriate action. We cannot reverse the changes that have taken place, but we can be better equipped to live in this world. We can change the consciousness of the world if we can change ourselves, and we can achieve this with a natural daily practice.

T'ai Chi, then, is not a flowing dance in an open field on a sunny day. It is a physical representation of the concept, theory, and way of Taoist philosophy as expressed in the *Tao de Ching*. Embracing this philosophy of nature through consistent physical practice transforms our consciousness. It enhances our well-being. Taoism guides us to adapt, and it provides a strategy for conflict. Without these qualities, we risk living as helpless individuals in a difficult period of our history. This outcome does not have to be, but avoiding it requires our effort and commitment.

SOMETHING
FROM NOTHING

A significant but often overlooked part of the T'ai Chi form comes just before the opening, when the individual stands still and quiet, not yet moving. This is called *Wuji*, the state in which there is balance and emptiness.

Once I became aware of the concept of Wuji, I was fascinated by it. In Wuji, all things are balanced in the void. There are no differentials, as a wholeness exists in this emptiness. Once you begin to move in the form, the positive and negative energies expressed as Yin Yang begin to exchange, moving from Wuji into T'ai Chi. This process very much resembles the cosmos and the Big Bang theory: the idea that the universe was caused from a point of nothing and out of it exploded positive and negative energies, continuously traveling and expanding through space and time—and we are all a part of it.

Before anything, there is Wuji. Even the Bible describes this process: *First there was the Word*. The Word represents sound. Sound comes from silence.

All new things—be it learning T'ai Chi, a new subject, language, relationship, or job—must first come out of an emptiness. Some people may perceive emptiness as desire, hunger, ambition, or lust, which characterizes it as a negative, feeble, or aggressive state. But emptiness is the beginning of opportunity. Simply understanding and appreciating that fact can change your attitude and understanding of your situation, such as the loss of a job, relationship, or home.

Think of it like this: Music can only occur if there is silence first. A painter can only paint onto a blank canvas. A writer can only start with a blank page.

Wuji is the blank slate, the uncarved block, the clear state of mind. It is the essential starting point. Everything that follows is a new creation. If you were to buy a house or an apartment, you would most likely begin with empty rooms. At this point the room exists without purpose. It is not defined, but it exists. It is only when you place objects in the room that its purpose begins to emerge. Add a couch and TV to make a living room or den. Add a large table and chairs, and it becomes your dining room. Add a bed, and it becomes a bedroom.

This Wuji state exists only momentarily before the T'ai Chi form, but it is developed through the practice of meditation. Meditation enables us to eliminate the noise and distractions that influence our perceptions, cloud our judgment, or make us respond in inappropriate ways. A clouded mind reduces our ability to use our instincts effectively.

Instinct is in our DNA, a natural behavior developed as a means of survival for ancient humans. It is informed through the five senses: visual, auditory, sensing and touch, taste, and smell. The body and the brain rapidly exchange information through the nerves and biochemical reactions to reach a conclusion and create an action. But instinct can be influenced, sometimes inaccurately, by perception, memory, and judgment. Developing a practice of freeing and clearing the mind enables you to perceive, process, and respond to new situations more spontaneously, accurately, and appropriately. We open the pathway for instinct to function without the ego or the interference of conscious thought.

A Wuji mind may very well be the fountain of youth. I remember when my niece was three years old. We were standing at the window on a winter day and snow began to fall. She had never seen such a thing! I asked if she would like to come outside with me and catch the snow on our tongue. I'll always remember seeing this child, so exuberant and filled with excitement, joyfully spinning with her head back catching this new thing—snow— which had never existed to her before that moment.

Children are filled with boundless energy and are mostly happy. They don't perceive obstacles. They don't fear rejection. Children run all around the house or yard picking things up, touching, tasting—sometimes making us cringe as they test the world. We commonly refer to kids as blank slates. Their minds are empty and not yet filled with stimuli, labels, and conditioned behavior bestowed by parents and grandparents, school, local customs or norms, and traditional and social media. The empty mind is clear, curious, and excited. The child's mind is a blank slate, but more importantly, it's energetic intelligence.

Adults can practice being empty and remaining curious, which keeps us excited about new things. We can experience that childlike energy and happiness. This mindset isn't something that can be instantly called upon when needed, though. Instead, think of it as a place that is easier to get to the more often you visit. It's like taking a long-distance journey. The first time might require a map, guide, or GPS. Things look a little more familiar the second time you make the trip, and after many trips you know how to arrive on your own. Your access to the destination—Wuji, emptiness—becomes easier to attain when you seek it more often.

Access to the Wuji state through meditation can be practiced as part of your daily T'ai Chi training or independently during another part of the day. You can meditate while waiting on a line, even if for only twenty seconds. You can take two minutes to meditate at your desk. Take ten minutes at the start and end of your day. Meditate on a train or plane ride. Or light a candle, put on some ambient music, sit on a comfortable pillow, and meditate for up to an hour.

With consistent practice, your mind begins to adopt a new way of interacting and responding to the stimuli generated from the outside world. You become increasingly resilient, adaptive, open-minded, flexible, and energized, because your mind has been less cluttered and regained the capacity to act as an instrument of thoughts, uninterrupted by memories that condition your thinking.

The Wuji mind moves into the T'ai Chi state with clarity, immediacy, and the ability to seek balance in the present.

Seeking balance is seeking wholeness. Wholeness is found in relationships. We cannot truly achieve wholeness in a relationship with a lover, family member, friend, or stranger unless we first become empty. Empty means the loss of "I," the ego, which creates division and fragments rather than unity. The loss of "I" means not seeking approval or appealing to disapproval, not acquiring a dominating power over others, and not seeking greater wealth at the cost of another. You exchange the reflexive drives of need, desire, and fear for a life of humility and a happiness free of burdensome calculations.

With the Wuji mind you see things as they are, not as you perceive them to be. The quiet mind will witness a mountain, an open sea, or a dramatic event without adding something that is not there. You hear a sound or voice without applying your own tone. The Wuji mind understands things through evident interpretation and isn't distracted by subtext, hidden meanings, or mysterious innuendo. You can walk your path undistracted and change direction only when your genuine circumstance permits or requires it.

This is what the *Tao de Ching* means when it teaches "doing without doing." The Wuji mind takes the conscious mind out of the equation, allowing the inner dialogue between the subconscious—the spirit mind—and the intelligence of the body to harmonize, communicate, and express itself through action as a complete being. The next time you play your T'ai Chi form, take a minute to acknowledge the Wuji state before you move into the Yin Yang exchange expressed through the form. The Wuji state is the real beginning of the T'ai Chi form, and achieving it is the genesis of an open and free-thinking mind.

Inspiration for Practice

KEEP THE MIND OPEN. We all possess different physiologies, experiences, and preferences. Stay open to another person's version of T'ai Chi, and remain open to your own version, which will be unique to you based on your own body structure, feeling, and state of mind.

How can the mind be opened? Through meditation. Sit in a quiet space. Focus on your breath, each time making the inhale or exhale smoother and longer. If a thought occurs, let it, and then return to your breath. Observe, but don't judge. When you don't impose a word, label, image, or pattern on thought or action, the mind opens.

YIN YANG
(IN THIN AIR)

I was once asked to present a class on the Yin Yang elements of T'ai Chi. This outdoor event would take place in a park nestled along the southern shoreline of Long Island, New York. I knew the attendees would be a combination of curious first-timers and experienced practitioners. I wondered how I would explain the Yin Yang elements within the T'ai Chi system, but also how Yin Yang applies to daily life. The answer eventually came by looking up.

I committed to the presentation and had two months to prepare. It seemed like enough time but proved to be not as much as I thought. I had just made a professional change and was acclimating to my new schedule, processes, culture, and systems. At the same time, a family member suffered complications in surgery and was in serious condition in the hospital. The Yin Yang of my personal and professional lives was not lost on me, but ruminating on this was low on the list of priorities.

Over the following weeks, I settled into my new role and had early successes with high visibility. The weather was beginning to warm, and I enjoyed walking to my Park Avenue office. At the same time, the health of our loved one became increasingly grave. The patient finally reached a point where, as the surgeon told me, "the next two weeks will determine life or death."

I'd been reluctant to offer anything that might have been perceived as detrimental or working at cross-purposes with the medical staff, so I hadn't offered any Qi Gong solutions. But at this point, I believed that I had nothing to lose. If this person were to pass, I didn't want to look back and feel that I hadn't at least tried to help. So I took the leap.

I took my family member through Qi Gong sets that I customized based on her energy level, physical capabilities, and ailments. I started simple and added more to each set incrementally. After a few days, the attending nurses reviewed her vital stats and told her to keep doing what she was doing—because it was working! This was the first step in a reversal of fortune. Qi Gong alone couldn't have changed her condition, given the severity of the situation; the expertise of the medical staff along with the sophisticated systems and machines of the hospital were essential for recovery. For a person at this critical stage, that cannot be overstated. The two combined, however, yielded the best results. Upon reflection, I realized that in addition to the physical attributes of Qi Gong, what may have been more important was that the patient, incapacitated for months, depressed, and demoralized, was now participating in her own recovery. Small successes like moving her fingers and toes quickly progressed to lifting her knees and then legs, and eventually sitting up and then standing up. Within six weeks she was home for a family gathering and slowly walking around the house.

A follow-up email about the upcoming T'ai Chi event hit me like ice water. The message confirmed that I was to present my Yin Yang class the next week. I hadn't thought about the content. I needed to pull together my presentation fast.

Sunday came and went. Monday passed. I decided that I could demonstrate Yin Yang in a Qi Gong breathing set, showing where it exists in a technique from the form and as a self-defense drill. All great, and all relevant, but I still couldn't think of an easily accessible, real-life example of the Yin Yang elements at play—until that Tuesday.

I was waiting for a morning train to Manhattan and turned to look at the sunrise over the trees. My eye traced the arc of a seagull and I decided to observe the bird's movement. It was here that I found my answer.

Watch a bird in flight, and you'll see it alternate between flapping its wings and gliding. The alternating of movement and nonmovement is a clear example of Yin Yang. But the action and nonaction that occur when a bird takes wing is a surface-level and simple example. The truth lies deeper.

Yin Yang is the symbiotic relationship that exists between all things moving through the universe. A bird alternating between flapping and gliding is engaged in a symbiotic relationship with the air. Observe how a bird moves its wings to rise or move forward and then lets its wings stretch out and rest while the air carries it. The bird may move its wings fast in the wind but then ride the current. The flapping enables it to travel a linear path and then yield to the arcs and turns of the air. The bird glides along, quickly flapping its wings for air pockets, then returns to a natural coast.

Watch any bird in the air, and you witness a dance between animal and element. The creature never fights the air but aligns with it. The bird is never concerned about reaching the destination or at what time, but arrives just the same. This was a revelation. The truth and beauty of Taoism—of Yin Yang—was alive right in front of me.

I delivered my workshop to a positive and open-minded group and I believe they were able to take home an exercise, concept, or approach that improved their T'ai Chi practice, even in a small way. Maybe one of them will begin to look up, or look within.

Yin Yang patterns exist all around us: hot and cold, night and day, winter and summer. Countries experience periods of peace or conflict. Companies experience high earnings or lower revenue as demand changes, which in turn is reflected by the ups and downs of the stock market.

These examples are extreme to illustrate a point. They seem like opposites but are connected by funda-mental connecting principles, which continuously evolve from one point to the next. Hot water becomes warm, then cool, and then cold, for example. Yin Yang exists in the closer proximities of your life, too.

Observe people around you. You may see one who has a new job or one out of work, one working excessive hours or one resting on vacation, one healthy or one dealing with illness. Over time you'll see their situation or condition—positive or negative—change. It may be a subtle change in the person's circumstance or thought process, but it is a change nonetheless. However overt or subtle, there *must* be a change in polarity, just like winter turns to spring and summer to fall. A person's achievements, losses, trials, or ordeals correspond to their beliefs, decisions, actions, and interaction with the influencing agents of progress and outcome. The Yin Yang symbiosis is the root of all things and the path of life.

Yin Yang also exists within us as a functioning part of our physical system. Breathing, for example, has two parts. An inhalation may be Yin, while the exhalation is Yang. If the person emphasizes one over the other, like the shallow inhaling and heavy exhaling that a depressed person exhibits, the breathing is imbalanced, which sets off a subtle but significant chain of health-related conditions that eventually become serious. For instance, shallow breathing limits the range of motion in our chest. The shoulders may eventually tighten and lift. This impacts the upper quadrant of the chest—the scapular girdle, where lymph nodes reside. The poor flow of lymph fluid could make the body more susceptible to several maladies, including lymphoma. The good news is that simple proper breathing can reduce or avoid these potentialities.

Try these three breathing patterns several times and make note of the effect:

1. Shallow inhale and heavy exhale
2. Deep inhale and shallow exhale
3. Even inhale and exhale

The first two can be very uncomfortable, and since this is an exercise, you may be exaggerating.

However, for some people these types of breathing patterns continue over long periods of time and become the new normal, and this new normal bleeds into our thought patterns, emotions, actions, and interactions. A person can become negative, angry, or depressed, which creates conflict or hardships around them, impacting relationships and their ability to function at work or in social settings. The person may turn to drugs or alcohol or engage in activities that further erode their sense of worth or self-respect. It seems like a stretch, but just look around.

The good news is that, like all things, this framing or mindset can change. The first step can be as simple as changing your breathing. Proper breathing methods can be learned by anyone at any time, and will have a profound impact on physical, mental, and emotion health.

The pluralism of Yin Yang is part of our broader lives, too. How many times have you heard about someone who hit rock bottom and then created a product, book, screenplay, or other innovation that catapulted them to great fortune? We tend to view the situation in an idealistic way, but consider this: the new idea materialized and was actualized when their life became empty of other distractions. Like exhaling and inhaling, emptying creates the next opportunity to become full.

We're viewing these life-changing events as being part of a simplistic process, but with the recognition that the path may be long and difficult. The point is to be able to look beyond a hardship with the knowledge that the condition will change at some point. It always does. We can keep our mind clear and focused on the flow of events and evolution of our process instead of being distracted by comparing our present situation with the noisy influence of opinions, labels, status, or personal aspirations. It isn't always easy, but this ideal is worth bringing to our life. Recognizing the distractions renders them empty and meaningless, enabling us to focus on responding to our present circumstance more fully.

Yin Yang concepts like full or empty are the foundation of T'ai Chi theory and practice. Beginner T'ai Chi students focus on balance and weight shifting early in their training, sometimes working through an entire form focused on footwork. Over time the student begins to understand how to place the weight on one leg while removing weight from the other, all the time maintaining balance and structural alignment. The Yin Yang of weight shifting is weaved into each posture within the form, developing one's sense of stability through varying positions. The lesson of this physical discipline is to learn to balance through constant change.

Changes in weather, government, the economy, and even our individual temperaments add up to a varied and unpredictable day, even for those living a life of apparent routine. Navigating these changes is best accomplished when you have a mind and body that is centered—a psychological and physiological "home base." It is our point of balance. From this place you adjust and flex to change—meeting a Yin condition with your Yang response, for instance—without losing your center.

Periods of personal or professional highs and lows happen to all of us. How we view these fluctuations influences our response, which impacts the outcome and how the incident is imprinted on the timeline of our life. Practicing the art of T'ai Chi empowers us to view our experience pluralistically from our center point, a neutral perspective that generates a more appropriate and resonant response. We make decisions based on our personal values and self-nature instead of being directed by outside influence. We are better able to live with the outcome and move on with less baggage.

Someone once defined a person with class as "not laughing too loud when they're winning and not crying too loud when they're losing." That elegantly describes a well-centered person who understands when a circumstance has run to its extreme and will soon return to the middle before swinging to the other extreme. It could be hours, days, months, years, or decades. Regardless, this type of person understands change as part of the bigger picture, allows it to occur, and then moves forward, like a bird in the wind.

Yin Yang Exists in Relationships

Ideal personal or professional relationships are based on each person complementing the other. They have different strengths that, when combined, compose a greater whole. But seeds of discontent may be planted if one assumes a greater portion of contribution with fewer rewards. The Yin Yang balance has then shifted too far in one direction. At home, it may be one person taking care of the house and children while the other enjoys time out with friends. At work, one manager may be putting out the fires while the other is creating political leverage to benefit themselves at the expense of the business. People who take more than they give or who unwittingly let the scale tip too far in one direction eventually pay the price. Over time, these people lose the benefits offered by the other. Their accomplishments eventually deteriorate and reduce to very little. They lose power. Their Yang energy becomes Yin energy.

Being mindful of the differences in the other person presents opportunities to grow in the space between you. The gaps or weaknesses you perceive in the other person are based on your strengths and orientation. But the other person can see you in the same way: their strengths are the lens by which they perceive your weak areas. The sword cuts both ways.

Instead of the tug of war between your egotistical drive to change another, why not recognize how the other's gifts can balance or enhance who you are and what you do? Your relationship is the interchange of Yin and Yang.

It is the harmony of opposites. Creating the ideal balance of power involves exposing oneself, so it must be rooted in trust but also in expecting the unexpected. It is how we grow together.

> *The Tao never does anything*
> *Yet through it all things are done*
> *If powerful men and women could center themselves in it,*
> *The whole world would be transformed*
> *By itself, in its natural rhythms*
> *People would be content,*
> *With their simple, everyday lives*
> *In harmony, free of desire*
> *When there is not desire*
> *All things are at peace.*
>
> —*Tao de Ching*, Verse 32

Reconsidering Our Approach to Living

Living a Yin Yang life pattern might seem counterintuitive to many of us. Western culture has evolved to celebrate intense drive and output. If you're not working hard, working out hard, striving, constantly busy, and always on the run, then the perception is that you're not doing enough. Or you're not "succeeding." A daily routine of high-intensity effort, output, and results can be depleting. It wasn't always this way.

The early days of the nation were built on trading and partnering to survive the new frontier. The seventh day was used to rest and to cultivate faith. There was a give and take, a Yin Yang of active and passive living. In the modern world, we're focused on business meetings, emails, and the like into the late hours of the night, motivated by the fleeting sense of satisfaction that we're keeping up with or passing everyone else. It has been labeled "work/life balance." But without the Yin Yang of active and passive periods, where is there balance?

This mode of living is draining. We're constantly emptying our well, the mental, physical, and emotional energy we must use throughout the day. Many people burn up their reserve energy. As our threshold of tolerance increases, the depletion is barely noticeable and becomes a new normal. It's only when crisis strikes—an event requiring our mental, physical, emotional, and spiritual resources—that we realize we may not have enough, if any, available. We are then left to deal with the crisis and its impact without these tools of empowerment. Now exhausted in life, we may be bulldozed by a traumatizing and life-altering crisis, while remaining powerless. Not arriving at the destination point as a participant, but as a victim.

We have within us the power to change this way of life.

You can mitigate the intensity of modern living by ensuring a daily practice of self-cultivation through T'ai Chi's hidden lessons on Yin Yang. When you have cultivated these resources, then you can meet a crisis and flow through change, even if it is difficult. Your choices and actions arise spontaneously and accurately. If the crisis is Yin, you may align (Yin) or counter (Yang).

Engaging in a form of self-cultivation elevates your level of consciousness, illuminating or creating awareness of the bigger picture. It becomes a system of faith. It feeds your soul.

It may be the nurse who studies yoga, the lawyer who spends the evening lost in creative writing, the scientist who seeks to understand religion, or the banker who learns guitar. The subject or interest is less important than the process. In my experience, T'ai Chi embodies all these attributes and is a place of solace.

T'ai Chi offers a philosophical, physical, mental, and spiritual center that is increasingly accessible through practice. Daily practice brings you to the source more immediately. The channel or passageway remains open and deep like a wellspring. Each morning I practice Qi Gong and T'ai Chi forms to synchronize mental and physical movement. I harmonize the conscious and unconscious, the body and the mind, the mind and the soul, the material and the spiritual. Opposites are balanced: Yin and Yang. In this unity there is power.

All things have a symmetry if you look for it. Learning, understanding, and integrating this symbiosis into our core nature is a way to evolve into an effortless but refined and higher state of being. Symmetry—balanced thinking or perspectives—can be developed and fortified through exercise as a physical ritual. T'ai Chi is among the most evolved and effective.

A person refining themselves through physical movement is like a sculptor chipping away at the stone to create smooth lines, curves, and balance. With T'ai Chi, you are chipping away at yourself. *You* are the work of art.

T'ai Chi aligns you with the forces of nature and in doing so connects you to nature in a deeper and more profound way. You learn the significance of change and how to flow with it while maintaining inner balance. The change in physiology from consistent T'ai Chi practice begets a change in perception, emotional stability, and a wider perspective.

You learn to balance the Yin and Yang within yourself and in the exchange between yourself and the world around you. Many of life's problems are reduced, solved, or accepted and then left behind as you continue to move forward, eyes to the horizon, with a heart glowing, emitting a radiance that is unconsciously noticed and sought by those around you who possess the same gifts but aren't yet aware of how to actualize them.

Inspiration for Practice

WHAT TO PRACTICE? Begin with the things you love in T'ai Chi and use that as your starting point. Then, with the guidance of your Sifu and your own inquiry, think about what you can develop to reach a physical, mental, or spiritual goal. Remember that they all interact—and the process never ends, so relax, enjoy, and love it.

NEW WORLD, OLD WAYS

*Bringing T'ai Chi's Ancient Lessons
to a Modern World*

"Technology has progressed more in the last twenty-five years than since the beginning of the history of man," an old friend said to me as we sat at the kitchen table, enjoying drinks on a sunny afternoon in late summer. We'd met through our kids and immediately became lifelong friends. He is a craftsman. I am more of an artist. We are different, but in a way that complements the other. We have differences of opinion in some areas but listen to each other. We exchange ideas and points of view. I learn a lot when we're together.

On this particular day, out of the blue, we began to discuss how fast humankind was progressing—in fact, doubling the progression with each new innovation— faster now than at any point in history. While it seems difficult to quantify this notion, I think back to landmark discoveries (fire, vaccinations, splitting of atoms) and inventions (the wheel, language, the printing press), each of which would take a century or more to develop, integrate, and gain mainstream acceptance. The current state of society reflects a profound acceleration of development that is prolific in opportunity and progress, but also fraught with hazard.

I think of the many big-budget Hollywood films that predict a time when robots will rule the world—or apes, come to think of it. (Okay, so it will be robots if we continue with technological discoveries, and it will be apes if we really screw up. For the time being, it seems like we are moving toward robotics, but I digress.) In these films we see that people have lost control of their destiny. They have developed a program, a system, or an artificially intelligent being that somehow turned the tables on humankind and will surely rule the world unless our hero does something quick. The challenges are mounting for the modern movie hero. With every new generation of Hollywood production standards, the villains become more terrifying, a chilling parallel to the development of technology.

Most of these movies are cautionary tales. I believe the writers are using their monsters metaphorically. The real "monster" is how technology is increasingly controlling our lives. The movie is an extreme representation of an outcome that has already begun to emerge. Just look around.

Have we become passive enablers, lulled to sleep by the ease of technology and a willingness to surrender a piece of ourselves for the sake of convenience or entertainment? It is a slippery slope. We must consider how much of the self is up for grabs. We're increasingly rely-ing on technology and social media platforms for infor-mation, facilitation, and validation. Our reliance is a tacit permission for the system providers to influence how we think and how we behave. It is costing us a sense of identity, self-worth, and the ability to solve challenges ourselves. The very engine of the most profound human progress has also been the source of the most significant human suffering. If the development and implementa-tion of technology is irreversible, then how can we pre-serve our authentic self?

The simple answer, at least for me, is to recognize tech-nology as a tool that a person uses to perform a job or achieve something. We control the tool—it does not con-trol us. T'ai Chi is not a tool, but more of an instrument. It is a prism by which we can understand our inner nature and corresponding values and beliefs, which can be man-ifested in the external world through tools like technol-ogy. We become empowered and sovereign. This is true freedom.

Each time I practice, it is a ceremony, a prayer in motion. A ritual where ego and pride are diminished so that deep-seated self-knowledge can surface. I am observ-ing the flow of movement as it occurs, with awareness of form as it unfolds, experiencing a cycle of change that connects like a golden thread throughout. There is a spirit of intent that must be sustained over the length of the form. Opening the organs, meridians, and ligaments, lengthening the spine so that Qi, the bioelectricity and biochemistry, flows unhindered and quiets the thinking mind so that the unconscious mind—the link to our spirit, our true nature—can dominate.

I listen for the messages and lessons encoded in the form by the creators, who had limited resources and no computers so incorporated their lessons into the art. The forefathers of T'ai Chi made their art a living document to teach us about nature and the universe. The practitioner who seeks this path will naturally assimilate these lessons beyond T'ai Chi to all the tools that are available, including the digital realm.

T'ai Chi training is based on Taosim and Ch'an Buddhism, with detachment as the root of the art. T'ai Chi masters won't cling to a novel device if it is not useful. They do not place higher value on something that has limited function or is purely for entertainment. They see it for what it is.

> *When the ancient Master said:*
> *if you want to be given everything, give everything up.*
> *They weren't using empty phrases.*
> *Only in being lived by the Tao*
> *Can you be truly yourself.*
>
> —*Tao de Ching*, Verse 22

History and Human Nature

Our history is an account of the periods of accord and discord, achievement and failure, composure and commotion, all in a constant shift. Nations, organizations, towns, families, and individuals will at one time or another experience periods of difficulty, no matter how much they attempt to mitigate risk or insulate themselves from these forces. Nothing is absolute, and there are no guarantees.

Remember that T'ai Chi and its underlying system originated during a period of dissonance. It was developed to meet a need. We must not allow the current dynamic forces to confuse us, nor seek permanent refuge through temporary satisfactions provided by high-tech entertainment. It's better to find a practice like T'ai Chi that will calm and empower us through these shifts.

History also tells two stories: one of the progression of humans and the other the nature of humankind. We have progressed beyond the imagination of our ancestors, and yet our basic nature has evolved very little in all this time. Our primal impulses, needs, emotions, rituals, cultural and social norms, and interactive behaviors aren't that different from what they were in centuries past.

Functioning in a modern world requires us to adapt to the new technologies without being diverted from the requirement to understand our own nature. Understanding our nature means accepting natural inclinations and instincts while learning to regulate them. Then we are better able to embrace change, discord, and progress without losing ourselves.

Understanding and cultivating your nature, then, won't happen by downloading the latest app. Instead, I propose a daily practice or ritual of T'ai Chi, kung fu, or even music, painting, cooking, and literature—ideally a combination of all. Engaging in each process helps us to understand ourselves and our relationship to the world around us.

As I studied and practiced T'ai Chi and kung fu, I learned that alongside kung fu, the Shaolin monks also learned and practiced calligraphy, poetry, music, and philosophy. Kung fu was a piece of the puzzle, part of a broader pursuit to understand and elevate the individual to the highest level of human potential. The modern kung fu master who only knows how to fight may have missed the point, in my opinion.

For the most part, technology is intended to reduce or eliminate tasks that keep us from pursuing more profound endeavors. Instead, technology's constant demand for attention will move us further from the self-cultivation required for true happiness and a meaningful life if we allow it. Technology has become a way to be more productive, but the expected level of productivity heightens with each upgrade. People are struggling to keep up, and it's at least in part because they're running in the wrong direction. Exercising a philosophy like Taoism through the practice of T'ai Chi can help steady our course.

> *The Great way is easy*
> *Yet people prefer the side paths*
> *Be aware when things are out of balance*
> *Stay centered within the Tao.*
>
> —*Tao de Ching*, Verse 53

Inspiration for Practice

FIND OPPORTUNITIES TO BRING YOUR LIFE AND YOUR ART TOGETHER. Everything you do influences your development. Look at how you can apply the T'ai Chi principles of movement, philosophy, and elements of health into your everyday routine. Think about how you walk, open the door, interact with others, view a change in circumstance, and unwind before going to sleep. Make a journal to record your thoughts, observations, and progression.

A PATH TO
EXCELLENCE

People often join a T'ai Chi class for health, social contact, or fun. Others begin lessons with set goals based on their perception of the principles, strategy, and form of expression that characterize the art. Even with different goals, learning the theory and applications remains the same. What goals can you have when beginning your T'ai Chi journey? There are many targets and milestones to reach, but the primary aim of studying a martial art like T'ai Chi is to begin a path to excellence.

A T'ai Chi novice may be attracted to the sense of peace, the dance-like movements, or the spiritual essence of the practice. Others might arrive at T'ai Chi seeking to recover from a surgery or to improve their health. Some people are referred to T'ai Chi training by physicians seeking to avoid drug prescriptions for common ailments or anxiety. The motivation varies but usually centers on one specific need in the beginning. Each person enters to satisfy that one need but in doing so has opened a doorway to the myriad benefits that come from

T'ai Chi training. A personal sense of quality and excellence is one of the greatest benefits of training in T'ai Chi and a recommended path, regardless of the original motivations.

When you begin to train in T'ai Chi, the first step on the path to excellence lies in understanding what the art is, what it offers, and what it requires. Misconceptions might cause you to give up on your journey. You want to be sure that you have the right instructor and that the style of T'ai Chi is a good match. It's also important to have a realistic sense of the time and effort required to learn the basics and to eventually master the art.

A qualified instructor should have at least ten years of training and experience teaching under the guidance of their *Sifu*, or Master Instructor. The teacher should understand the history of the style, its theory, Qi Gong sets, the T'ai Chi form, Pushing Hands drills, martial arts applications, and weapons. A more advanced Sifu will possess knowledge of herbology, acupuncture, and deep tissue massage. Most importantly, the Sifu will be able to communicate the art and respond to your questions with clear and comprehensive answers. The best Sifu possesses a deep understanding and teaches it through experience and explanations.

There are five main styles of T'ai Chi. They are branches from the same root theory and history of T'ai Chi, but each possesses distinct elements of style that may appeal to you based on its aesthetics and your physical ability. For instance, Chen style, developed by the Chen family, is the mother of the T'ai Chi system. Chen T'ai

Chi has deep stances requiring leg strength and includes stomping and explosive techniques.

Yang Luchan was the first outside student the Chen family agreed to teach. Yang mastered the system and, realizing the Taoist essence, went on to study Taoist yoga, which he combined with the Chen style to form Yang T'ai Chi. The Yang style is expressed in a form that is soft throughout, slower in tempo, and larger in movement. If you have ever seen people practicing T'ai Chi in the park, then you've probably seen the Yang style.

If low stance work isn't suitable, you may seek the Wu Hao style, which developed from Chen and Yang combined and is characterized by slow but smaller movements and a higher posture. A second Wu style exists, which is defined by its hand form, weapons, and Pushing Hands drills.

Of the five styles, Sun style places the greatest emphasis on gentleness. Because it is less vigorous, it may be best for older students or those with physical limitations.

Some people fall into hidden traps if they ignore the quality and content of the art, dismiss the Sifu's instruction, or lack commitment as a student. There are students who unknowingly invest years with a poor teacher, for instance. Some students are collectors, bouncing from teacher to teacher to learn one or two forms, then moving on with little more than a surface understanding. Then there are a few who believe they've mastered the system after six months or a year and view themselves as an authority, possessing greater knowledge than their teacher. While it might have been gratifying at the time, none of these people have uncovered the hidden route of discovery that leads to the genius of the art.

It's not all their fault. The common thread among these types of students is their short-term thinking, which is supported by a media-driven society heavily conditioned by advertising gurus. Watch any commercial for an exercise machine or workout facility, and you're bound to hear the words "fast and easy" at least a few times. Fast and easy is attractive. It is seductive. It's fun! Fast and easy is appealing because people are so busy and focused on attaining perceived success (seemingly enjoyed by everyone around them) that they have been unwittingly robbed of time for physical development, and even less for self-cultivation.

In the right T'ai Chi classes, you'll meet people who possess a genuine desire to develop a high level of skill. These students are consistent in attendance, practice on their own, constantly ask questions, and may seek additional information by reading books or blogs. They are willing to invest their time to reach their highest goal. And they are rewarded for the investment.

Learning a sophisticated form or to fight at an artistic level opens the door to the timeless wisdom of life, which is a source of solace even in these modern times. T'ai Chi offers strategies for your moments of alignment or conflict—psychological or physical—in your place of work, home, or on the street. T'ai Chi remains vital, and a source of vitality, because regardless of the progress of humankind, human nature remains the same.

* * *

Bodhidharma (AD 448–527), a holy man born to a Brahman king, traveled from India to spread Ch'an Buddhism in China. His message was that wisdom, the highest attribute, is achieved through the perception of self-nature. To Bodhidharma, material offerings, even the temples and statues constructed by Chinese royalty with holy intent, were inferior. They were symbols of holiness but not themselves holy.

When I read the story of Bodhidharma, I realized how the priests, monks, and prophets of the ancient societies all preached against prioritizing objects over the higher aesthetic of a life realized through self-understanding. It is a lesson that we can easily relate to, even if we lack knowledge of Chinese history, because the same lessons exist in the West, where religions like Christianity share these tenets. For instance, the second commandment handed down by Moses is "You shall not make idols." The first commandment is to "Have no other gods before me." Bodhidharma and Moses are essentially preaching the spiritual over the material as essential to rising beyond the difficulties of life. Internalizing these values through a practice like T'ai Chi is a significant step toward a better quality of living.

Bodhidharma arrived at the Shaolin temple and observed the monks' lack of physical fitness and inability to concentrate for extended periods. After spending nine years meditating in a cave, the Ch'an Buddhist priest returned to introduce unifying mental and physical exercises so that the monks cultivated their Ch'i (pronounced "chee") energy, thus increasing concentration and achieving enlightenment—a personal relationship with the nature of all things that is understood but cannot be conveyed through words, symbols, or material objects.

As Ch'an Buddhism began to spread, Taoist priests became intrigued, as it aligned with their own philosophy of a higher mental and physical existence. For Taoists, *Tao*, or "way," is the universal natural law, expressed with mutually opposing forces of Yin and Yang. Aligning with these forces will result in achieving *Te*, or power. Taoism's master treatise, the *Tao de Ching*, states: "Know the masculine (active principle), but keep the feminine (passive principle)." Balancing the two in accordance with nature enables the practitioner to respond to life spontaneously, a principal goal in the practice of Chinese martial arts like T'ai Chi. The ultimate goal is to flow with life and respond to conflict with a resolve to restore the life flow.

Unfortunately, a better *quality* of life is often mistakenly pursued through *quantity* of life. We live in a consumer-based society that encourages the acquisition of more goods and services. It is what keeps the US economy moving and the country thriving, theoretically for the good of its citizens. But is accumulating more things necessarily best for us? Have these material offerings distracted us from self-understanding? If each new gadget, device, object, or toy (adults have toys, too—think jet skis) represents a new layer that covers our essential nature, is it possible that we are burying ourselves alive?

It seems to me that many have prioritized the creation over the creator. They have focused on material representations rather than seeking and cultivating an understanding of themselves through the interchange of Yin and Yang, cause and effect, the origin and expiry that occurs in the movement of life. But it's never too late to change course, as many of us do at one time or another.

Learning to play the T'ai Chi form with smooth, continuous movement takes time and patience. As Oscar Wilde said, "The art is to conceal the art," and T'ai Chi masters make incredibly complex movements seem effortless. One of the key goals of practice is to eliminate and reduce any nonessential movement. This is the "smoothing out" of the body, which opens the pathway for better flow of Qi energy. In this art, we learn through a process of reduction that the individual actually gains greater economy of motion, and with it comes clarity, energy, health, and power. Less is more. Over time, this principle becomes a key to deciding what is essential and nonessential to you. Quality eclipses quantity.

The result is increased mobility and freedom to move through life in a healthy mental and physical state while liberated from the trappings of maintaining status— professional or personal, with the accompanying financial debt and stress.

The T'ai Chi student begins to learn about the calm, patient consistency needed to build proficiency. This process mirrors nature, which is quiet during creation and noisy only in destruction. With this understanding it becomes clear that daily practice, with its corresponding ups and downs, ultimately elevates the individual's level of skill. They just may not see it right away.

* * *

I'm always amused to see the face of a T'ai Chi student at the six-month to one-year mark. They often say that they feel like they haven't achieved anything yet, until they see a new student, contorting and struggling, just as they had only six months before. Recently a second-year student learned to turn and step from one posture into the next and remarked, "That would have taken me three weeks to learn a year ago!"

The culture of almost any T'ai Chi school is welcoming and nonjudgmental. Anyone who has studied for a year or more is familiar with the challenge of learning to coordinate the mind and the breath; then the mind, breath, and body; and then the mind, breath, and body united in action through postures, forms, and drills designed around conflict. The experienced student recognizes their own struggle to achieve a level of proficiency, so is only happy to help.

Beginner students will also see that development does not follow a linear trajectory. This dynamic exists everywhere, from the cardiogram to stock market charts. By accepting the ups and downs that exist in all things, the individual has a broader, pluralistic perspective that exists beyond "times are good, so I am happy, but if times are bad, I am unhappy." Instead, the ups and downs become part of your whole existence, making for a more complete and fulfilling life.

For those who dedicate themselves to fully learning T'ai Chi, the benefits are manifested into everything we do. We discover the enjoyment at the beginning of something and let it flourish over time instead of rushing to reach the end. We come to appreciate the process as it unfolds and celebrate the small, subtle details experienced along the way. The need for instant gratification or rushing to the end evaporates, and with it, the frustration we experience when we're focused on the fool's gold of future outcomes instead of the jewels contained in the present moment. Like the performance of masterful music, the art of T'ai Chi transforms the process of living into an experience where the point *is* the experience itself.

Of course, even with this new perspective, there will be challenges. Challenges must exist in order for a person to grow. Challenges make us focus. It is from that focus that we learn and grow as people because we're essentially striving to master the situation that exists for us. That's right: the situation that exists *for* us. This situation or challenge is an opportunity for us to create and grow as human beings. The tools to meet that challenge, whether trivial or life-threatening, are cultivated and developed through a daily practice of T'ai Chi. Our mission for learning T'ai Chi is to break from the status quo and inspire a new perspective of values, priorities, and balance in our life.

Developing and cultivating skill in T'ai Chi means developing philosophical, health, and defense skills that can be applied to your life. It is an art where you can achieve an overall sense of excellence—a quality in being—regardless of income level, mode of living, or station in life. It just takes practice.

Inspiration for Practice

PRACTICE LIKE A MANTRA. A mantra is a word, phrase, or sound that is repeated again and again, especially during prayer or meditation. Take one piece of the form and practice repeatedly, until you've forgotten what or how you're moving. It becomes its own living thing. Note how you feel and try to bring that to your total T'ai Chi form.

WHY IS T'AI CHI
SO SLOW?

Slow is smooth and smooth is fast.

—NAVY SEALS MAXIM

There's a YouTube video of a satirical televised T'ai Chi sporting event. Two announcers introduce each T'ai Chi master as they enter the ring. The match begins, and each contestant engages in painfully slow movements, delivering unobstructed blows that have crippling impact. It is hilarious. It also illustrates how most people perceive T'ai Chi only as a slow-moving practice. Then there's the classic image of an elderly person practicing, reflecting another common misconception of T'ai Chi. For people in the West, the message of this image is that T'ai Chi is something you do when you grow old. They have missed the point. What the image suggests is that you can grow old and still be vital and healthy *because of* practicing T'ai Chi.

Why do people assume that something isn't effective just because it's slow? The theme of slow and steady has been embedded in our culture from childhood, when we first hear the story of the tortoise and the hare. Remember, a tortoise can live up to 150 years. We learn this valuable lesson, but then forget. We grow into adults and enter a profession, marry, buy a house, and start a family. This is a good life. The danger comes when the family gets sucked into the vortex of "keeping up with the Joneses."

This costs time and money. Maybe Mom will go back to work. Dad takes on more work. They run the kids to all the latest popular activities. They have acquired money and material, but where is their life? The family jumped on the hamster wheel and now needs to keep running. All of this to keep up with the pace of life they perceive as successful.

Now, what was the point of that story they read to their kids? Is it possible that slowing down in our exercise, our thinking, our way of life, can have a positive impact on our health, well-being, and quality of life? The answer is yes, and in more ways than you might imagine. You might even reconsider the allure of keeping up with the Joneses.

Slowing down is a step toward good health. The first and most important lesson of T'ai Chi is learning to relax your body, which is easier to do when you practice slowly. You begin in a relaxed state and then add only the amount of tension needed to perform the movement. The goal is to open the channels and pathways for better aerobics and circulation to allow flow of Qi, the intrinsic energy that exists in all living things.

The concept of relaxation for health is discussed in Western medicine, but many people misinterpret the advice to mean "sit on the couch." T'ai Chi begins with teaching you how to move while in a relaxed state. The slow pace enables you to pay attention to the areas of tension and release it. Over time this process becomes automatic. You purposefully move while consistently adjusting to smooth out obstructions, which creates the fluid and supple motion in T'ai Chi. Over time this becomes ingrained into common physical movement.

Think about your veins and capillaries as garden hoses. When a hose has a kink, the water has trouble passing. If you extend the hose and remove the kink, the water flows. The process of removing physical tension from your body "unkinks the hose" of the veins and capillaries, which increases circulation and nourishes the internal organs, enabling them to function properly.

T'ai Chi involves a sophisticated series of steps, turns, and twists that are coordinated with a variety of movements with the hands and arms suspended in the air. Each posture within the form creates a physical tension and release within the body, which opens the pathway for Qi circulation. The slow tension and release create a tourniquet effect, similar to yoga.

Take, for example, a vital organ like the kidney, which functions to remove toxins from the body by processing up to 1,700 liters of blood each day. Parts of the T'ai Chi form will use the muscle located at your back to exert pressure, which stimulates that specific organ. The pressure constricts the passage of blood, so it "backs up" or builds in the system.

As you release out of the form and into the next, the muscles slowly relieve the pressure, allowing blood to flood into the organ with greater velocity, which cleans and replenishes. Think of it as internal power-washing. Most people improve their health by working out, but they focus only on muscle. While this does prevent loss of muscle mass as we grow older, it doesn't guarantee sustaining power. Additionally, these individuals are doing something healthy while ignoring the more critical need to take care of their organs. People rarely die from muscle failure, but many die from organ failure.

Daniel Reid writes on this extensively in his book *The Tao of Detox.* In it, he describes how diseases and degenerative conditions that had previously existed only among the elderly are becoming more prevalent in the younger population. Reid explains how pollutants, poor diets, drugs, and alcohol have overloaded the body and its natural detoxification systems. While many people believe that they are improving their level of health through "hard sports" like football, weightlifting, or running, they're actually increasing lactic acid and carbon dioxide in the bloodstream. The book recommends T'ai Chi and Qi Gong, as it pumps lymph through the system and increases the free circulation of blood without lactic or carbon dioxide buildup. Toxins are drained and eliminated without physical damage to the body.

* * *

Documentaries on high-performing athletes will inevitably reveal the hours of demanding training that the athlete invests over days, weeks, months, and years. What is seldom included but nonetheless critical is the time the athlete spends watching footage of themselves. Every high-level athlete does this. They watch for proper form and alignment, arcs and integration, steps, turns, twists, and swivels to achieve a fluid and powerful performance, the highest potential of the human physique. But to really examine and correct the nuance of movement, they must view the footage *in slow motion.*

Practicing the T'ai Chi form is the same as watching a slow-motion video performance of yourself. The procedure was created at a time when moving pictures weren't even conceivable, yet the goal was identical. Moving through the form slowly enables the T'ai Chi practitioner to trace the flow of each movement, thus removing tension, burrs, and obstructions. You make corrections in real-time slow motion.

Practicing slowly allows you to focus on the feeling of the movement and the physiological effect it has within your body. Some people feel the impact immediately. Others may take more time to orient their attention internally. For them, the focus is usually more from the outside in—using outside events to influence thought or focusing attention on the musculature rather than ligaments or tendons, for instance. One isn't better than the other, but the ultimate goal is to balance the two. It might take more time for an externally oriented person to experience the inner effects of T'ai Chi. Once they do, they'll possess a more holistic perception of their physical being.

The Yang T'ai Chi long form is recommended for both slow and fast practice. The goal is to slow the form enough that it is complete in one hour, or speed it up to complete in less than five minutes. Both are very challenging, and each enhances the other. The slow, relaxed, and consistent movement creates muscle memory of the most efficient pathway. The body moves in concert with itself. When sped up, this form maximizes its potential to generate power.

Practicing the T'ai Chi form slowly also removes physical stress. It opens blockages and enables the body to function as a complete system. T'ai Chi elevates health and increases longevity because the body is nourished without wear and tear. The slowness enables you to monitor and make corrections to each movement to ensure proper alignment and maximum performance. The body functions in its optimum state.

Calm the Mind

For the last twenty-five years I've followed the same morning ritual, although at first, I wasn't aware of why I went through it, only that it felt right. I rise early to spend an hour on Qi Gong and practice the T'ai Chi form and isolated techniques. I commute by train while reading a book that will teach me something. I take time to meditate. Finally, on the walk to my office I listen to music. A scientist might study this approach by measuring each level of brain activity, but to put it succinctly: I awaken the body, awaken the mind, and raise my spirit. It all starts with my T'ai Chi practice.

The slow, smooth physical movements of T'ai Chi are excellent for the body but also beneficial for state of mind. For years people have referred to Eastern-based health as *mind/body* systems, a label that suggests the two are separate. Quite the opposite: the mind is connected to the body through neurological pathways and biochemicals that transmit intelligence; sensory information is sent from our nervous system to the brain and messages are sent from the brain through the spine to generate a physical response.

Changing physiology, then, will alter the messages sent to the mind. If the nervous system senses a state of calm, then that message is sent directly to the brain, which in turn will remain calm, the opposite of a "fight or flight" response. The brain waves, which are related to our state of consciousness, will adjust.

In *The Body Electric*, authors Robert O. Becker, MD, and Gary Selden break down the frequency of brain waves into different levels of states, including delta (.05–3 cycles per second) at the level of a deep sleep, theta (4–8 cycles per second) at a trance or drowsiness, alpha (8–14 cycles per second) as relaxed wakefulness or meditation, and beta waves (14–35 cycles per second) for everyday conscious activity.

People today rise from a delta or theta state and seek to modulate directly to beta as the dominant frequency, usually with the aid of caffeine. At the end of the day, many people watch television programs with intense drama, violence, or sexual content or focus on the stressful challenges related to work, bills, childrearing, or relationships, all while maintaining that beta state. They then retire to bed and struggle to relax down through three levels of brain activity to achieve a peaceful night of sleep.

In this scenario the alpha and theta states are almost non-existent. Instead, these people are forcing the dominant brain cycles to modulate up and down by as much as 10× capacity to function in the extreme, ignoring the midlevel states that are essential for healthy brain function.

Is it possible that people on extreme ends of the brain wave cycle, such as a depressed person who sits around the house or sleeps, or the classic Type A person who is overactive and stressed out, exist on the fringe because they're not able to regulate the proper level of brain wave activity? Having a system that can adjust the brain cycle up from delta or down from beta to achieve a "middle ground" for brain activity may actually enhance their overall mental health. Practicing T'ai Chi in the morning, at midday, and in the evening, even if for only twenty minutes at a time, in effect applies moving meditation to modulate up from morning drowsiness or down from the stress-inducing challenges of everyday conscious living.

* * *

Slow practice enhances the function of the mind and increases concentration. Practicing T'ai Chi slowly requires a higher level of focus and presence. Slow practice transitions consciousness from the outer environment to your inner environment. It's not as easy as it appears.

In the poem "In My Kitchen in New York," Beat writer Allen Ginsberg describes his thoughts while practicing T'ai Chi in his apartment. Ginsberg's mind shifts from the form's posture to items on the refrigerator. Every new posture triggers an observation in the apartment, sparks a memory, or forecasts future activity. He even thinks about not thinking and getting back to T'ai Chi! One thing is for certain: Ginsberg's poem communicates how easy it is to be distracted away from the inner sensations experienced during the form.

Regardless of intelligence or experience, focusing purely on your form at a slow pace is extremely challenging. Think about it like this: you're expressing a long series of subtle, sophisticated movements with your limbs moving in seemingly opposite directions at a pace slower than anything you've ever done, while totally relaxed, oh, and by the way—don't think about anything else. As soon as you think about something else, the connection is interrupted and you've removed the intent, which is the point of the process, because slowing down and focusing on each moment trains you to be in the flow of life.

In *The Art of Happiness at Work*, the Dalai Lama and Howard C. Cutler, MD, discuss the state of *flow*, a concept developed by psychologist and social scientist Mihaly Csikszentmihalyi. A person who is in flow is completely absorbed in what they are doing, fully present and engaged as their skills are being summoned to achieve a desired goal. Buddhist psychology calls it "meditative stability." The Dalai Lama goes on to say how many ancient spiritual rituals include practices to stabilize the mind. A stabilizing meditation could be a spiritual chant or reciting the rosary. It could be crocheting or practicing a musical instrument, as Sonny Rollins famously did on the Brooklyn Bridge. It is most certainly present in the practice of slow T'ai Chi. The slow-moving meditation and underlying Taoist philosophy that are the root of T'ai Chi provide meditative stability.

In fact, this practice creates a deep level of concentration that will influence how you perform at work, prepare a meal, or even rake leaves. It teaches patience and a calm persistence to pursue excellence while resisting the need for immediate satisfaction. It allows you to actualize and fully express yourself, in the moment, attentive in the flow of life.

Slowing down counterbalances against the pace of society.

It brings focus back to what is essential.

Slowing down allows us to perceive.

It reminds us to return to an attitude of letting things flow naturally.

All of which can make us feel happy and fulfilled.

Inspiration for Practice

HOW SLOW IS TOO FAST? You should practice as slowly as it takes to execute your movement perfectly. You are practicing slowly to maintain relaxation and to slow down your brain activity. Practicing slowly establishes and maintains our synaptic wiring. Your brain will fortify the connections so that the integrity of the motion is intact at faster tempos. You are training to increase focus, and to focus your intention.

IS T'AI CHI REALLY A WORKOUT?

At one time in my life I was a scrawny kid. It was a period when I felt weak and uncertain and awkward. It was also the time I deemed myself a lover, not a fighter. I was never built for fighting, anyway—never had the physique. But when you're a kid, "might is right" tends to dominate the social landscape, so developing a large physique was advantageous. Still, I never wanted it.

This decision can make you vulnerable to intimidation. At the time I didn't realize that there was a different way to develop my physical self. It took me a quarter century to understand the difference between strength and power, fitness and health. The difference between chasing a well-defined shape and attaining wellness.

When I was fourteen, I went to the home of a girl I liked and wanted to date. I was nervous and very self-conscious. Her brother, who I knew, let me in. He left the room, and she hadn't come down yet. I sat quietly at the kitchen table, observing the afternoon sun on the azure-painted walls, the dishes in the sink, the cheap knickknacks randomly placed on the shelf, the ticking of the clock, the remnants of salt on the Formica table.

The back door swung open. The brother's friend let himself in, looked around, saw nobody but me, and decided to take a seat. I didn't know him but knew his reputation. At seventeen he was the quarterback on the high school football team. Everyone called him the Incredible Hulk because even in high school the guy was tremendous. I tried to act cool in the summer heat.

He looks at me. "Who are you?"

I mumble my name, trying to avoid eye contact.

"What do you play? You play football?"

"Who, me? Nah, not really."

"You lift?"

"Not really. . . . I'm . . . a drummer."

"What? You're in *drama*?"

I remember how different I felt from him and others at the time. We could not have been more opposite from each other. Eventually I realized there was nothing wrong with me, I just chose a road less taken. Over time I realized that I was on the right path.

I have never been a jock or gym monkey. I could never see the appeal of lifting weights in a room filled with people working out. I don't condemn their choice; it's just not for me. I have an active mind, so I need to be mentally engaged during physical activity. I wasn't aware of that distinction in my teenage years.

Over time I learned that I prefer training for skill as opposed to working out. I want something that conditions the body but enriches more deeply than what is attained through physical activity alone. I did eventually realize that martial arts made sense for me. Through the training and conditioning, I discovered that there is more than one way to work out and the immeasurable benefits that come from training properly. I can be healthy and powerful without becoming the Hulk.

* * *

With T'ai Chi I'm not just exercising but learning and developing a higher level of skill and a deeper level of understanding. Understanding of my true center of gravity. Learning to be grounded, or rooted, to achieve balance through stepping strategies. I am training to move in any direction: up and down, right and left, forward and backward.

The directions are refined and encoded into foundational techniques like *Peng* (expand/ward off while moving up, down, or to the side), *Lu* (roll back to yield), *Ji* (press forward or inward), *An* (stamp down, forward, or upward), *Cai* (grab up, down, diagonal, or sideways), or *Kao* (bump forward, downward, or sideways). I develop and refine the ability to coordinate complementary but sometimes opposite movements (Yin Yang) between the upper and lower body, left and right sides. I am building strength in the legs and back. I am understanding power by training my body to move as a single unit.

Each week you learn, build on, and refine body movement while strengthening its connection with the mind. The mind controls movement and interprets perceptions received through touch, sight, and sound. The stronger the connection, the faster the transfer of information. The mental and physical align in movement. The body changes: it becomes more supple and fluid. The muscles tone and tighten but remain flexible. The physical benefits of body sculpting exist, too. They're not the primary objective, but a byproduct of effort directed toward these other goals.

* * *

In early stages of T'ai Chi training, the emphasis is on relaxing the muscles in order to develop the tendons. The next stage conditions and tones muscles through constant coiling and uncoiling, which creates twists in the limbs and core. The twisting and untwisting of the torso massages the vital organs, enhancing their function and improving overall health. Unless diagnosed with muscular dystrophy, people rarely die from muscle failure, but, as noted earlier, many of us will die from organ failure. This reality should motivate us to seek systems of wellness that do more than just build muscle.

The deep stances and constantly shifting footwork condition the leg muscles. Suspending the arms strengthens the back and shoulders. The bones react to the pull of the muscles and tendons by building more cells, which, because of the breathing techniques, are more oxygenated and becoming stronger. T'ai Chi focuses on softness so that these benefits can be maximized. Dedicated practitioners are eventually introduced to advanced techniques for muscle development. Weight is added, mostly in the form of weapons like sword or staff, which are introduced once the student has mastered open hand forms. This is advanced-level T'ai Chi training.

You can achieve good health with modest goals in early training. As your level of health increases, you may naturally move your fitness goal. Your body condition will become your guide as you explore more advanced training.

* * *

T'ai Chi training contains its own Yin Yang element. The Yin of T'ai Chi is spirit, intent, and Qi (energy). The Yang of T'ai Chi is the physical dimension and body movement. T'ai Chi trains you how to use the Yin to direct the Yang. But the art has been taught from a purely physical, or Yang, point of view in the past.

According to T'ai Chi legend, Yang Cheng Fu's father only allowed his son to teach forms, focusing on the movement without intention. He had a specific reason, though. This type of training took place during a period of Chinese history when families, villages, and schools didn't share their secrets with any outsiders, thus preserving the knowledge for their own protection.

Training the form without the Yin element is still done in some modern schools. It may provide a "workout," but as the body ages and muscle mass decreases, the need for spirit and intention becomes more critical. It is a sustaining element that T'ai Chi continues to develop into our advanced years. Training to use intention as the motive force of energy reduces excessive physical effort and concentrates your energy into efficient action. This is a key to longevity.

* * *

One time my Sifu told me about his Sifu, and how their teacher/student relationship began. It was not unlike the beginning stories of other traditional martial artists. It went like this: each day my teacher, Sifu Kaparos, would visit Chan Tai San at his apartment in Brooklyn, New York. Chan would have Gus hold a stance, doing nothing else. Once Gus became too tired to maintain the stance, his lesson was over for the day, and he was sent home. Eventually Gus held the stance for an hour. Then his training began.

At the surface it seems that Chan was testing Gus, to see if his dedication was at a level where it was worth Chan's time and effort to pass on his knowledge. I'm sure that was part of it, but I now realize that this wasn't the full story. Chan was conditioning Sifu Kaparos before the training started. *Zhang Zheng*, or the Tree stance, is one of the oldest—if not *the* oldest—forms of training in Chinese Qi Gong. Practicing this form opens the channels and meridians. It conditions your legs, arms, and back muscles. It aligns the nervous system, increases circulation, and calms the mind. It is at once the simplest exercise and yet the hardest to do.

One only reaches the point of holding the Tree stance for an hour with consistent effort. You must also have a vision beyond the exercise. You must realize that the pain and discomfort have a benefit, and focus beyond them. The concentration must be on the long term, because eventually you condition yourself beyond the discomfort and reap the benefits.

And why not? After all, what's the rush? If you could go back in time to anything you had started to learn—dance or baseball, for instance—and had the time to really focus on the fundamentals, those beginning steps, would you do it? The answer is yes, I'm sure. Because with those fundamentals firmly in place, your overall level of performance is that much better. Too often people feel the need to rush to the end, as if learning were a race. They reach their imagined finish line, declare themselves a master, and then move on to something else: collecting the martial arts, or any endeavor, with an illusion of achievement and success.

True masters master the basics. They focus on the minor details, smoothing out the lines and creating better efficiencies. Master T'ai Chi practitioners recognize that superb basics create a strong foundation for continued growth. Their foundational skills can be expanded and applied in a variety of ways. The person who invests the time to develop deep roots will master the style of T'ai Chi they're learning but will also be able to learn, adapt, and integrate other styles.

The true long-term health and wellness benefits of T'ai Chi require an investment of time. The student must learn to calm themselves through breathing and meditation, then learn the basic stances and hand positions, then movement, then forms, then applications and weapons. Unlike a gym, where the commitment is in the form of membership, T'ai Chi asks for sustained effort from the student, who is also learning and refining themselves while they work out.

Over time and through repeated practice, questioning, and testing, students will adopt the techniques and philosophies of greatest value while discarding those that, although valid, may not be appropriate or useful based on their individual physiology and philosophy. The changes may be major, even groundbreaking, but more often are minor variations. This process is essential. It's what keeps this art evolving and alive.

Learning and development takes time. Mastery requires time, commitment, and effort. Kung fu is literally translated as "excellence through hard work." You can attain kung fu in your T'ai Chi.

Of course, not everyone will reach the master level. A large percentage of people aren't interested in pursuing T'ai Chi to become a master or an instructor. They just want to train enough to be healthy and happy. And that's really quite enough. The goal is your own. Seek the level that is right for you at this time in your life. If anything, try to project forward a little to determine your level of health over the next five or ten years and set a goal based on how you want to feel *then*. It could help. In any event, we all share the common goal to do our best.

Training in T'ai Chi will bring results, but you may not see them right away. Slowly chipping away at the form, with your body moving through strange and complex new movements, can be frustrating at times. You feel awkward and weird. But observe how you begin to move during the rest of the day. Your step, or the way you enter a doorway or move in a new direction, will have a quality that didn't exist before. Eventually that quality will exist in the T'ai Chi form; it just takes more time because it isn't common movement. Achieving quality requires patience—not just for results, but with yourself. Recognize that you're making deep and lasting changes at the physical and mental levels. This cannot happen overnight.

We all learn at a different pace. We listen to our instructor's words and see different images and make unique correlations and connections. So, my version of the T'ai Chi form will inevitably look different than yours. My learning curve may be long (it is, by the way), but maybe, once learned, the technique will never have to be retaught as it typically will for fast learners. Patience, persistence, and perseverance are required for real development. But remember to also keep it fun.

It's helpful to know how you train most effectively, and also to understand that your approach will be different than those of other students. You want to be a good training partner when in a group class. Occasionally students who train together clash during lessons. It usually plays out like this: one student has more serious goals than the other and may be a little further along in their training or understanding of the art. They will watch their training partner struggle with a technique. Out of frustration, they'll begin to correct or criticize the less experienced person. Even with good intentions, this approach helps no one. It is *not* fun.

If you're an advanced student, help only at the request of the student or your Sifu. If you're a student in need, communicate what you don't understand or if you need time alone to figure it out. The goal is for everyone to reach their own potential at their own pace, regardless of whether it's a weekly workout or a daily path to mastery.

* * *

During the summer months I like to eat breakfast outdoors on my back deck. I hear the birds and can see the sun slowly rise. Add a vegetable omelet and hot cup of coffee, and life is heaven on earth. One morning, and for each morning after, a bright light flashed in my eye. It was so bright that my eyes would immediately shut for protection. I thought nothing of it the first day; I'd even forgotten about it until the same thing occurred the following day. I realized a pattern on day three and tried to figure out the source near the end of the week.

The light was blinding because it reflected the sun. The flash was unpredictable and instantaneous, so I couldn't wait for a specific time and then trace the source. I would need to wait for this flicker of light and then look around. So, I waited.

There it goes again.

I stood up and walked the perimeter of my yard. I saw a small child, maybe three years old, sitting in a little swing on the raised deck of a home whose yard joined my property at the southeast corner. The child was making happy baby sounds and playing with a stuffed animal and a mobile. The child's guardian, an older Chinese woman, was also there. She was moving in smooth circles, arcs, and turns and then the light hit my eye again, reflected off the blade of her sword. I watched in silence that day and for weeks after. The lady was a grandmother. She would bring the baby outside and then practice Qi Gong, the T'ai Chi open hand form, and then the sword form. Then she would stop and play with the baby.

I noticed that this woman practiced without placing any special emphasis on what she did. She didn't treat the T'ai Chi practice as something exotic. She didn't seem to care if she was watched. She didn't compete. The woman didn't see herself or her practice as unique. It was her own form of wellness. It was just something she did—a way of life.

Inspiration for Practice

CREATE A FRAMEWORK AND SCHEDULE FOR YOUR PRACTICE. You may emphasize stances one day, Qi Gong another day, and a difficult section yet another day. You may do the form or applications. You may freestyle. The key is to set a structure that aligns with your goals and vigor, but occasionally break the structure so that it doesn't become routine.

HOW DO YOU
DO IT ALL?

*T'ai Chi's Symmetry and
Influence on Multitasking*

T'ai Chi appears simple when you see the form presented by a master. The movement is fluid, the tempo is even, and they have a calm expression on their face. The form is a beautiful art, expressing physical potential while possessing the attributes of a poem: a composition that strings together imagery to create an overall sense on the surface, but also reveals an intricate and deep internal structure with multiple meanings. Like the adage says: "Still waters run deep."

Those who have attempted to copy or mimic the movements casually or during a class usually find themselves contorting and unable to move their body to match what they've just seen. In fact, some individuals become twisted like a pretzel, caught up in themselves like a fly trapped in a spider's web. For the teacher, those early attempts by the student provide insight into their frame of mind and their integration of the mind and body. It establishes this person's unique starting point.

Regardless of point of origin, it's fair to say that we all start at the same general place, which is confusion. I know I did. I found it difficult to keep track of what my hands were doing, but also the legs and feet, the position of the hips, the straight spine, and oh, by the way, don't forget to breathe. Sound familiar?

Over time the guidance of a good teacher, combined with your own patience and practice, will begin to yield results. You will come to understand how positions move in complementary opposites to create a symmetry, albeit in a strange posture that seems to lack any meaning or function. But it is a symmetry nonetheless.

Understanding this symmetry of movement is the first opportunity to connect with nature. Through time and evolution everything on this planet has developed a structure that is self-stabilizing while aligning with, or balancing against, the powers of nature with the least required force or effort. Honeybees, for example, create complex structures for storing their honey. You might expect that the bees create round space within the honeycomb for maximum storage. In fact, they build hexagons, which require less energy to build but offer maximum storage capacity. Bees are just one example of the many forms of life that favor a more intelligent labor system. It works best, and it fosters longevity.

Perfecting physical symmetry and mental balance is a lifelong pursuit. It is also one of the things that keeps us coming back to T'ai Chi. Because even with daily practice, some part of the body will be slightly out of alignment, or the footwork won't quite coordinate with the hands, or the movement gets ahead of the breathing. . . . And so, we try again. Which is okay, because the imperfection is itself a part of nature.

In nature there are no straight lines. The next time you're outside, use your eye to trace the branches of a tree. Look for a straight branch. You won't find one. Yet the tree is beautiful and unique, certainly different from the trees right around it, which may be of the same species and from the same seeds. This little exercise is a great meditation and nice reminder of our own strengths, imperfections, and uniqueness.

Learning the T'ai Chi movement with the correct symmetry requires a great deal of concentration. But it is relaxed concentration, which is developed through still meditation. While relaxing with focus on the breath, you'll develop each movement of the form like learning a word, and then piece the words together to form a sentence and eventually a composition.

Try this simple meditation while standing or sitting:

1. With a straight back, lower your chin as if your head is held by a string at the crown.

2. Place the tongue on the roof of your mouth.

3. Relax your shoulders.

4. Relax the lower back and then the hips.

5. If you are standing, bend your knees slightly.

6. Pay attention to your breathing.

7. Begin to shape your breath into long, even, and focused inhalations and exhalations.

8. With each breath let the body settle and relax, creating a feeling of heaviness.

Your mind will naturally drift, so let it happen. The key is to let the thought occur and then return your attention to the breath.

Try this for three, then five, then ten minutes each day. Eventually you will begin to feel a physical and mental shift. Continue to practice until you can meditate for an hour daily. It could be at home but just as easily in a park or on a train, plane, or bus.

The benefit of this level of concentration can easily transfer into daily living, whether it is studying for an exam, working to a deadline at work, or simply spending time with your family. Training in T'ai Chi is more than physical discipline. It trains a way of thinking. Absent is the tense and frenetic monkey mind that impedes your thought process and distracts from what you're actually involved in doing. Instead, you channel a calm focus, which increases efficiency and maximizes results with less effort. Just like nature.

Leveraging One Technique for Multiple Applications

The complexity of each shape in the T'ai Chi form demands the practitioner's full concentration, which strengthens focus and slowly reveals multiple internal patterns. Each movement is improved over time as one learns and becomes more proficient at coordinating their body. With continued practice the mind increasingly sends clear messages to the legs, waist, torso, and arms to move in directions that seem to oppose, but actually balance, the form of the movement. These early lessons are centered on physical coordination, which at first seems to be complex multitasking. The real lesson is that each position of the form is multipurpose. It contains multiple meanings, which change like facets of a diamond viewed from different angles. The content and meaning change based on how you apply the technique. In order to learn the form properly, you must adopt this concept, which can be bridged to areas of your life beyond T'ai Chi.

Each shape within the T'ai Chi form looks pleasing to the eye but can be hard to describe. Even a student with a fair amount of experience is challenged to describe what the shape is or, more important, why or how the technique evolved to its current form. As with all great art, the meaning is concealed, only to be revealed when a Sifu guides you in breaking a posture into smaller parts that each contain a specific purpose.

You will better understand the meaning of the movement by learning the applications. Over time you'll learn how the form is adapted to strike, push, pluck, rend, bump, or press. You'll learn hidden kicks and strikes, and see that strikes don't come just from the hands. You'll learn throws and joint locks. Suddenly a new world is revealed!

The brilliance of T'ai Chi is in how its creators were able or determined to consolidate an average of 10 distinct self-defense applications into each piece of the form. T'ai Chi as a system comprises approximately 37 movements depending on the style, and out of those movements there are at least 250 self-defense applications. No one person has completely unlocked and mastered all the techniques, so we're not sure if 250 is the maximum. There may be more.

Understanding and becoming proficient in the multiple applications within each posture of the form requires time and practice. From that practice comes a deeper understanding of and fuller appreciation for the depth and breadth of the art. It also develops a certain sensibility for synchronizing around your center.

Your attentiveness to the diverse applications emanating from a single position will increase when you understand the spiral points encoded within each posture. There are multiple applications because in T'ai Chi your spiraling point relative to the axis—your center—determines the function. This way of thinking can be applied to your T'ai Chi and presents opportunities for better efficiency at home or work. You can begin to learn how to maximize return on effort with simple tasks.

Let's say, for instance, you have a file that needs to be delivered to a manager on another floor. Delivering that file requires that you stop or complete your current task, leave your desk or office, travel to the stairs or elevator, arrive at the next floor, go to the office to drop the file, perhaps discuss the content for a few minutes, take the elevator back to your floor, return to your work area, sit, and then—and this is important, too—re-engage with your own work, which means reviewing what you'd been focused on or what was to follow next. If you assign a reasonable length of time to each event in this process, you'll quickly understand how much actual time you've lost for this extremely minor task.

But let's assume that the file must be delivered and that you have other items on your to-do list. With a little forethought, you may be able to maximize return on effort during the trip. This time when you take the file and begin to walk to the elevator, you stop by a colleague's office to follow up on something agreed upon earlier that day; as you pass another manager's office, you offer a short update on a project you're working on for them; and as you near the elevator, you drop off your outgoing mail at the reception desk. On the way back to your desk, you pick up a package of printer paper, stop at the restroom, and replenish with water, coffee, or tea before settling back in to the task at hand.

That same travel loop that was used to accomplish one thing now has allowed you to satisfy seven different demands with only a fractional increase in time. Once back at your desk, you can more fully concentrate on the task at hand because several others have been addressed.

Accomplishing more with less effort like this becomes addicting because it's more satisfying and less taxing. It can even be fun. And although it's widely known that the mind can't focus on two tasks at the same time, an unobstructed mind will be able to group, organize, prioritize, and execute more in less time. The key is to not get lulled into thinking you can do more and more.

When Yin Becomes Yang: Knowing When You've Gone Too Far

Teaching basic weight shifting drills or a technique like Brush Knee to a beginning student is an opportunity to point out a basic and important physical consideration. As the T'ai Chi student moves toward the finish of the move, settling into a Bow and Arrow stance, for instance, I remind them to be sure the knee doesn't pass the toes. Occasionally it might and there's no harm in that, but when it's done repeatedly the added forward weight neg-atively impacts the joint and over time can cause some real problems.

If we're analyzing the Brush Knee as a self-defense application, the considerations are more practical. Oftentimes the beginner delivers the strike but worries that they won't connect, so they lean forward toward me, their opponent. Their knee is now well past the toe. This is an easily exploitable position: the student's weight is fully committed forward, so a slight pull from me will bring them forward, off-balance and surprised. Their Yin has turned to Yang.

This person's powerful and effective technique, although executed well, quickly dissolved simply because they overextended by a matter of inches. To the classic T'ai Chi wisdom on fighting techniques, "Never chase the opponent," I might add, "Know when you've gone too far."

This lesson applies to balance and knowing when you're chasing something to the point of creating an imbalance. That pursuit may occur in fighting or in your personal and professional life. An effective, organized multitasking genius can easily trap themselves by taking on more, and more, and more. We can get seduced by our own effectiveness, piling the commitments up so that we're no better off. If you give yourself a minute to reflect on what has been accomplished and what remains outstanding, you can eliminate the tendency to overcommitment and get caught off-balance.

The Portable Health and Fitness Program

T'ai Chi is an excellent stress-reducing exercise, especially if you're a busy person with competing priorities and a lot of responsibilities. Of course, stress-reducing exercises can be found in many settings, but it might be difficult to access those programs. And while a gym membership has obvious benefits, I find that many people who have one can't seem to make it into the building. A person who learns T'ai Chi is providing themselves with a mobile fitness program that can be used in any place, at any time.

I've been able to practice in my office when on a phone call that doesn't require writing or even a lot of concentration. I've practiced on the top deck of a cruise ship at sunrise. I've practiced in my hotel room. And I can go beyond that hotel room. I have consistently found space to practice in New York, Los Angeles, Washington,

DC, Boston, Nashville, Philadelphia, Miami, Atlanta, Chicago, Athens, Zurich, Geneva, Dublin, and other cities. Most of the spaces I find are picturesque—hidden discoveries that I would have never experienced otherwise.

The discipline of meditation and practicing the forms of T'ai Chi transforms your home, work, school, hotel—any place you are—into a sacred space. That sanctuary, the consecrated place, can then be brought anywhere with you. Because it is you, by way of your daily ritual, who has created it. No matter what the demands of the day are, you can return to that place, because you maintain constant access.

Practicing in public takes some getting used to, but after a while you'll become comfortable and just get started. People generally ignore me, but some watch and enjoy it, as if I have become part of the attraction or a form of local entertainment. Once, when I had finished the form, I received a round of applause from two women visiting from China. They appreciated that I had the respect and commitment to study an art from their country. Other times, people think I'm a New Age hippie freak. And I'm fine with that. Those people move on with themselves and I can just do what I came to do.

Once, while in Los Angeles, I was walking back to my hotel after a long day of business when I was approached by a man who looked to be about twenty. He explained that he was a college student who had been in the park earlier and watched my morning workout. He then asked me what it was that I'd been practicing. I explained and then gave him a free first T'ai Chi lesson: standing in the post position for a morning meditation. The student had been stressed out over his workload and the performance pressure of college. So, my morning practice raised awareness of the art, which potentially changed one person's life for the better, even if only in a small way. In the spirit of multitasking, the practice achieved more than one goal that day.

> *Few will have the greatness to bend history itself, but each of us can work to change a small portion of events, and in the total of these acts will be written the history of (each) generation.*
>
> —SEN. ROBERT F. KENNEDY, Cape Town, South Africa, 1966

Inspiration for Practice

MAKE YOUR SACRED SPACE. Spend some time creating an environment that will help you return to the ideal physical, emotional, and mental state of being. Think about light and space. What will your eyes see? You may add photos, flowers, soft light, or candlelight. What scent helps you break the routine of the outer world? Incense or scented candles can help. What to hear? Add sound that returns you to that special place or that will mask sounds coming from other sources. It can be as simple as ocean or meditative sounds. It could be classical music or jazz ballads. I like rhythmic music. Experiment until you find the combination of elements that bring you to your own sacred space. You will eventually cultivate a sense of being that exists wherever you go, where every place you are becomes your sacred space.

"NOTHING SEEMS TO UPSET YOU"

T'ai Chi's Impact on Emotional Balance

My family and I were staying at the same hotel as our friends and their families during a springtime soccer weekend getaway. I was up early to find a place to warm up with Qi Gong and practice T'ai Chi before meeting the group for breakfast. I stopped at the front desk to ask about a park or someplace nearby to exercise. There is always a place to practice.

The concierge sent me to a tiny area of park hidden at the edge of town. We must have driven right past it when finding the hotel. The park was just a little walkway wrapped around a tree, with two benches facing a brook with a gently flowing three-foot waterfall. Perfect. It was a sunny and warm day in a relaxed small town, so I enjoyed some practice and made it to breakfast at the restaurant on time.

The kids were already wide awake and gathered at the restaurant ahead of their parents. We found them trying to balance saltshakers on the table and laughing. They were excited to be away together. Most of the parents began to amble in. They were still groggy, needing their first cup of coffee. So they sat, tried to make polite conversation, and waited for the server to come.

The server took our order and disappeared to get the coffee. Time passed. More time passed. One of the parents began to voice displeasure, which segued into a critique of the school her kids attended. Other parents interacted and voiced an opinion, but our friend only responded with sharp criticism.

Next, our friend questioned the decisions about plans for the day, when and how they were determined, asking, "Why couldn't it be done this other way? Shouldn't we have done this other activity instead? And where is the coffee? I can't function like this."

Our friend brought the dark cloud over her table of friends. Within a span of about ten minutes, this person's chronic pessimism changed everyone's attitude. When breakfast was served, most of us ate in silence, paid the check, and returned to the hotel room to prepare for the day.

A few days after our trip, I received a call from one of my friends with an unexpected question.

"Can we get together? I want you to show me what T'ai Chi is about."

Of course, I'm happy to share this amazing discovery with a friend. In fact, watching someone light up and become happy or excited when they discover this art is gratifying and fun to observe. We set a day and time to meet, but I had one question before we hung up.

"I'm happy to show you what I've learned, but I'm curious. I didn't expect this call. What piqued your interest?"

My friend told me that after the weekend, he and his wife had discussed that breakfast. At one point she said, "You know, our friend brought everyone's mood down, but I noticed that her sourness didn't impact Bill's mood at all. Nothing seems to upset him."

My wife would disagree. The reality is that we all experience—and should allow ourselves to experience—the full range of our emotions. To ignore or suppress them is unhealthy. However, the range, depth, and duration of the emotional response can be managed, shortened, and balanced within the broader range of the emotional spectrum. So, I still have my days.

That said, I have never met a depressed T'ai Chi person.

For me, and roughly four million others in the United States, T'ai Chi represents a thought process introduced and developed through physical exercise and martial applications to reveal a philosophy of life. A more holistic and pluralistic perspective emerges, and with it, the frenetic drive to chase down every problem diminishes. The need to control every situation is reduced because it's viewed as part of a larger pattern created by your actions (karma) and the reactions of those around you. By training in T'ai Chi Chuan, you internalize resilience, which in turn enables you to address the unique challenges of your life.

Among the greatest benefits of T'ai Chi is its capacity to help you manage emotional swings to experience a brighter, healthier outlook. Attaining an emotionally balanced state begins with training to develop physical and mental relaxation, then learning to maintain that composure when the training intensifies. By practicing to understand and master the T'ai Chi form, you metaphorically experience life's continuum and your perspective evolves from dualism to one that is more holistic. You acquire a greater self-knowledge, a sense of empowerment, and personal sovereignty. As a result, events and circumstances have less emotional impact on you.

It's often said that if you have your health, then you have everything. It has become a well-worn phrase because it's true. Problems will always arise at home, at work, and within your personal and professional relationships, but you can't address any of them if you're sick or hospitalized. For the person lying in a hospital bed and critically ill, life's problems become diminished. Their attention has shifted from what author and former CEO Dov Seidman has termed "way-of-life problems" to "end-of-life problems."

Faced with the potential reality that all may be lost, a terminal patient would willingly take back their life, problems and all. Now enlightened, they realize that even the problems are part of the fabric of their life. These problems are for the most part manageable, and some may even force change as life goes on.

You've seen this notion play out in several movies, where the main character, suddenly aware of their impending demise, begins to see life anew and swears that they will live a better and more fulfilling version. Off the movie screen, people make the same vow. There are those who take up a cause and become a symbol of change. Others take stock of their lives and are grateful for the chance they have been given, even if their lives can be messy at times. Then there are those who spend time pursuing their passions or life-affirming activities. Some change their lives permanently, while others slip back into their former selves within two years of the trauma.

There are some people who appear to be physically and mentally healthy, but never recover when setbacks occur during their life. Instead, those little demon problems gather and grow into towering monsters, dwarfing the spirit and reducing the will. I used to speak frequently with Susan, a beautiful, statuesque banker whose career and marriage became tumultuous. I would listen to Susan and try to offer perspective or support, but I now realize that it was without fully understanding her view of the struggle. After losing touch with her for thirteen months, I was heartbroken to learn that Susan ultimately took her own life.

Questions about Susan's action surfaced for me daily, but none more than *Why?* After some time, I realized that I could only try to learn from this situation. Susan's last act must have something positive or a ray of light attached to it. So, after much introspection, I realized my lesson: Life will change and sometimes in ways you don't want. You can choose to embrace it or may need to just accept and live with it. But above all, no matter how dire the situation seems to be, *keep walking forward,* because in time you'll reach the other side, even if the outcome isn't what you envisioned.

Life is always moving and so requires movement.

You can create a change in how you relate to life without requiring trauma as the catalyst. Beyond most exercise systems, training in a discipline like T'ai Chi strengthens your personal constitution. It provides strength from a center, especially when you enter periods of darkness and uncertainty. Learning a physical skill that is based on the ever-changing interplay of Yin and Yang promotes a healthy sense of sovereignty and perspective. It creates a reservoir for energy, willpower, and the spirit. And while you may not see the need to build such a reservoir based on the perceived arc of your average life, remember that life is unpredictable. The order of things can reverse in a moment. You may not yet possess the tools to address the specific problem, but a healthy mental and physical foundation is an ideal place from which to start. And change can begin with a simple shift in perspective.

"There are two sides to everything," the saying goes, and it is rooted in a truth. Day/night, hot/cold, left/right, clockwise/counterclockwise, up/down, in/out, and on and on, infinitely. How we perceive the two sides can make a difference in our view of the broader world. In the West, we tend to apply a binary view: 0 **OR** 1, black **OR** white, right **OR** wrong, good **OR** bad, half empty **OR** half full. An Eastern view is more pluralistic; each element corresponds with the other. Think of it as a complementary alternate or corresponding opposite.

One cannot exist without the other, so if one moves to the left, eventually they must move to the right. A world of only left-led movement doesn't exist. With this in mind, viewing a situation becomes less about the absolutes of: "It must be this or else it is certainly that." "It is only good or only bad." This thinking may create comfort or a feeling of security, but it is not universal intelligence, nor is it truth.

Placing perceptions into a fixed state provides an illusion of control—the idea that we have command of the situation, the will and power to manage or change it. But the real power exists within the person who does *not* attempt to reduce things into absolutes but rather perceives how the event is woven into the broader fabric. For example, a baseball player may be upset that the game was rained out, while across town a farmer is grateful that the crops will receive much-needed water. A holistic perspective embraces the opposites and provides a base or center—a place of neutrality—as things change.

Developing a broader, more objective, and less discriminate view of the world enables you to see patterns of nature—including human nature—and flow with it. For example, you may perceive changes in behavior among your managers that allow you to better anticipate upcoming changes in the company, even if you're not completely sure what those might be. When an announcement is finally made, you won't be as surprised as others who never perceived the change and who might be blindsided, upset, or even traumatized if the change is extreme or counters their perception of stability. Although you won't be able to change a situation that is inevitable, your perspective, emotional stability, and clarity of thought—free of distracting external influence—will empower you to make decisions consistent with who you are as a person. That is where real power exists.

* * *

Some people like to learn the T'ai Chi forms and a little Qi Gong and they're happy to have just those lessons. I encourage students to take the additional step to learn at least one application for each part of the form, simply because it enables them to better visualize and understand the martial purpose of the movement. A surface-level awareness of these techniques is sometimes enough for the student. But more often than not, the student becomes intrigued, then fascinated, and then obsessed with the applications. It's fun to teach, too.

Learning the T'ai Chi self-defense applications, the mid-range fighting techniques and close-range strategies that are developed through Sticking Hands and Pushing Hands drills, creates a sense of empowerment. This is a whole new world for someone with little or no fighting experience. To them, a fight—and in some cases, any level of conflict—is very stressful. Lacking tools of self-defense forces the person into a fight or flight response. They might cave in on themselves or just submit to the attack. They may build themselves up to a full head of steam and then lash out. This may be a passionate but inappropriate response and oftentimes makes matters worse.

Developing fighting skills, then, is more about obtaining a set of tools for the levels of conflict inherent in all situations. It is a method to elevate self-confidence in the larger settings of your life. It also develops a thicker skin. It instructs you on how to win and lose, which is a regular occurrence during the ups and downs of life.

I once had to spar with my older training brother, a bald and heavily tattooed man with a compact build. His day job was doing demolitions for a construction company, and he played in a heavy metal band at night. Everything about this guy was destruction. I stood across from him and prepared for the inevitable. And it came. I was completely overwhelmed and easily defeated. At first, I was deflated. I felt low and worthless. But then a day or two later, I realized: if I could stand across from a guy like that, even knowing I was in a losing situation, and still not back down, then facing someone outside the school, no matter how big they are, is no longer intimidating. I learned how to enter conflict without the fear of losing. This is a profound change in mindset that will permeate every area of your life once you experience and internalize it.

Most people lack the skills or actual power to truly dominate another person. Instead, they rely heavily on intimidation. But what happens when that doesn't work? That person rarely has anything left. And they know it. If you have ever stood across from them, remaining calm and unaffected, then you've engaged in the conflict by adopting martial arts' most common tenet: the art of fighting without fighting.

In our binary world of zeros and ones, you can view the conflict situation this way: if your opponent is negative and you remain positive, the dynamic is clear. If this same person is negative and you allow yourself to become negative too, then the situation changes. Now to win, maybe you decide to intensify your attack. But in doing so, you may become more negative than your opponent, which in relative terms means that they now have become the more positive party.

Remember that everything is relative because everything is related, even when in opposition. There is an interplay that will change the dynamic of the relationship within the exchange. A trap like this can be avoided if you practice responding to a negative influence with mental and emotional balance, as I was able to do during that breakfast.

T'ai Chi Chuan contains hundreds of applications and can be taught to students at any age or skill level. Even those who want to avoid sparring and potential injuries can learn the techniques and practice with little or no impact. This level of training doesn't guarantee complete control or safety, but the investment of effort can improve your odds during a physical confrontation. It will also help during verbal conflicts and with those who attempt psychological attacks, which often leave deeper and longer-lasting scars. Training to be effective in physical contact requires the right mental approach to be successful. You are using physical techniques to develop and improve mental strategies.

This feeling of empowerment, when taught correctly, also comes with responsibility. Protecting the weak, responding to someone in need, and, more importantly, understanding to respect and preserve life in all its forms are all part of the ethos of a true martial artist. Stepping on a spider in the house becomes a thoughtless and selfish act. You are destroying a life, no matter how small or insignificant. The empowered T'ai Chi person will lift the spider, maybe with a piece of cardboard, and place it somewhere outside the home. This small act is selfless and connects you with all of life—the *grand ultimate*, which is the literal translation of the word *T'ai Chi*.

The respect for life also extends toward all people (even those who oppose you), regardless of their age, gender, income level, profession, or station. By issuing respect, you gain respect, oftentimes even by people who don't personally like you. You possess power because you have mastered yourself instead of trying to master another being.

If you should enter into a conflict with someone, respect is important, maybe even more important, after the event. Every great document on warfare strategy includes the need for a plan of war, but also a plan for peace. If you knock someone down and the conflict is over, then offer your hand to help them up. At a minimum, walk away. Never humiliate someone who has been defeated.

This fighting spirit extends beyond individual conflicts to the ups and downs that make up the broader arc of your life. These are the daily battles we all must fight. And those daily battles will never go away, because it is part of our survival. Struggle is a byproduct of conflict. We struggle to work, earn, advance, improve our opportunity for happiness, and provide the same for our families. We find ourselves competing with other professionals to obtain work, striving to "get ahead" in the company, paying the bills, and yearning to be remembered as a great provider for the children, which can range from supporting them emotionally to providing financial support into adulthood, from driving them between activities so that they can explore every interest to flying them to exotic vacation locales to expand their horizons.

On any given day this person may view their personal situation as a success or a failure. It is a perspective that may be formed from past experiences or present circumstances. The focus may intensify based on the severity of the situation. The person's perception of how it plays a role in their broader life narrative becomes blurred.

During periods of difficulty, a person's response may range from minor irritation to frustration, anger, or despair. It can be difficult to live through a significant hardship and maintain some level of objectivity and a balanced attitude. I say "balanced" rather than "positive" here for good reason. In my opinion, it would be at best challenging and at worst disingenuous to experience a real struggle and be able to somehow completely rise above it. Maybe there are some people who can do it, but I'm willing to bet that the mass majority feel differently, myself included. That said, having awareness of objectivity and balance through daily practice creates a path forward from the extreme emotional reactions to intense life events, good or bad, more quickly. Life may knock you down, but you learn to get back up. Resilience.

By not trying to pretend things are great when they're clearly not, you remove a layer of unnecessary attention and mental focus. It's like shedding a thin layer of skin. It enables you to focus on the problem at hand without wasting energy on effort to promote an attitude that doesn't really exist.

At the same time, you needn't waste so much energy on despair. Focusing on the impact of the problem and how it affects your own life draws attention away from the problem itself and places the spotlight on you. That is called *drama*. You become your own distraction. Focusing on yourself compromises the attention and energy that could be fully directed at solving the crisis instead. Your situation will linger, you will feel worse for it, and a cycle has been put into motion until you (or your circumstance) change. T'ai Chi training is learning to avoid the drama by being a master of change, not a victim of it.

The meditative elements of T'ai Chi allow the mind to relax enough to widen the lens of perception. Pushing Hands drills and sparring exist as representations of the interplay between Yin and Yang—positive and negative forces, attacks and counterattacks, cause and response. You will win some and lose some. Just like in life.

T'ai Chi training ingrains a perspective that is peaceful, unwavering, and constant. It instructs us how to interact or relate without judgment or false expectations. You are focusing energy on the specific problem at hand—that reality of *what is*—without having the need to judge. You take yourself out of the equation, removing the ego with its useless commentary, to focus purely on action. You give the problem full attention until it reveals an answer or solution, which animates your response. This is the meditation of life. It is living in truth.

When some people see things as beautiful,
other things become ugly
When people see some things as good,
other things become bad
Being and non-being create each other
Difficult and easy support each other
Long and short define each other
High and low depend on each other
Before and after follow each other
Therefore the Master acts without doing anything.
And teaches without saying anything
Things arise and she lets them come
Things disappear and she lets them go
She has but doesn't possess
Acts but doesn't expect
When her work is done, she forgets it
That's why it lasts forever.

—*Tao de Ching*, Verse 2

Finding Yin Yang in Your Timeline

The following exercise adapts your life's timeline in a way that will show the plurality that exists. It is simple to do and can be fun while also aiding you in viewing your life with a broader perspective.

Take a sheet of paper and draw a horizontal line. Place vertical bar lines on the horizontal line in even increments. Place a number over each bar line to represent your age in five- or ten-year increments. Now take time to think about each period of your life. Place a dot above the line for positive experiences and below the line for negative events. It could look like this:

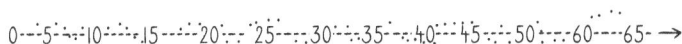

0--5-⋅-⋅10⋅-⋅-⋅15----20⋅-⋅25---30-⋅-35--⋅-40⋅-⋅45-⋅-⋅50⋅-⋅-60----65- →

Once you have completed the timeline, go back to the beginning and connect the dots, like this:

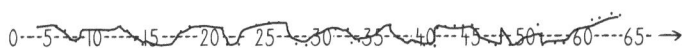

0--5--10---15---20--25--30--35--40--45--50---60----65- →

And then, pick an area, above or below the timeline, to shade in.

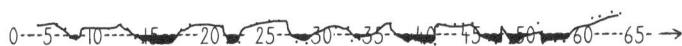

0--5--10---15---20--25--30--35--40--45--50--60----65- →

Notice how the events on your timeline aren't always above the line? Similarly, the timeline isn't filled with purely negative events. For the most part, the timelines I've created with my students are balanced, because nobody has it all good or all bad. Both exist and both *must* exist for one to live a complete life. Notice how the above-line events are white, while the below-line events are black. Do you recognize the Yin Yang pattern here?

Bonus: Look back at your timeline. Focus on the negative event as a starting point and ask yourself: How did this struggle or conflict move me into the next direction? How did I respond? Did my response lead to the next high point? How? When did Yin become Yang?

Using a timeline in this way presents an opportunity to view the big picture when it comes to your own life. This larger view of things can be helpful as you enter the darker periods of turmoil, upset, or tragedy. If you connect the dots, as we have here, you'll recognize that as time goes on, your life continues to change.

For many people, the confusion lies in the seemingly random and nonlinear unfolding of events. They fail to understand how a high point may contain the seeds that lead to a low point, or vice versa. They view these events in isolation, so they're often blindsided, never anticipating what could happen. To invoke a martial arts or boxing term: that person is caught *flat-footed*.

So, if we recognize and understand that life events will constantly appear above or below the line in varying increments, where is the constant? Look at your timeline again. Look at the numbers you placed on the bar lines. Look all the way across the years and at the far-right side, at the end of your timeline. Draw an arrow there. The arrow belongs there because your life is expected to continue.

And that is your constant. Your life is your constant.

The highs and lows of the timeline are the distinct Yin Yang of your life. You, and the life you live of choice and circumstance, are at the center. It is the signature of your life. Developing your life as the center—creating the stillness that is often described prosaically, but never defined or explained, by New Age and self-help gurus—is what enables you to recognize, move beyond, or even accept a change in circumstance. This approach seems antithetical to most people, who attempt to contain their lives by controlling each situation or each other. They scatter back and forth in a nervous panic, trying to plug each hole in the dam, all the while questioning the quality of their life, even if on a subconscious level. But the progression of your life is the center of all life events. Sometimes that means letting go of or accepting the things that occur.

The person who is calm and centered recognizes their own nature and so accepts the events as byproducts or results. Your response, with clear intent, becomes part of the pluralistic fabric, which changes the occurrence from one of conflict to one of interplay. Anything else, such as the loss of a loved one, is beyond our control. What is in our control is the time we spend (the center line from our timeline) with that person while they are present in our lives. And so, while we may mourn the loss, it can be with less regret.

Once again, we have a Yin Yang pattern of:

- **Yin:** Actions we take leading to results that form the ups and downs of our life over time; and

- **Yang:** Events that are beyond our control and therefore will occur whether we want them to or not

Knowing that both dynamics of life exist, why waste time worrying? It's better to spend your days cultivating an attitude and approach that equips you for those shifts, be they subtle or grand. While allowing situations to develop and play out may leave you feeling powerless, the reality is that by allowing the situation to unfold without intervening, but responding as it flows, is empowerment. The *Tao de Ching* says:

Mastering others is strength,
Mastering yourself is power.

Note that the word *others* is not limited to people.

* * *

During the fall season I begin to integrate a Qi Gong set into my private warm-up and at my students' lessons. One piece of the set, which can be done while sitting or standing, is called Circle the Wind Lasses. Picture the motion of your arms rowing a small boat. You inhale while circling the arms back, flexing the chest like a bow, inhaling at the beginning of the revolution and exhaling on the return. Do this twenty-four times and then reverse the motion for twenty-four cycles. The exercise loosens both the muscles surrounding the lungs and the shoulders, which stimulates the area of the body near the chest and shoulders that contains lymph nodes.

This Qi Gong set is followed by additional forms that were created to expand and strengthen the lungs. This makes sense to do as we enter fall, because the change in air quality from warm and humid to cool and dry affects the physical body. That change is first experienced in the lungs. Aligning the body with the change of season provides better health and well-being, which supports a positive attitude.

Integrating seasonal Qi Gong sets into your practice is an opportunity to align with the cycles of nature. The psychological effects of the season have been studied and documented, so suffice to say that with an elevated awareness you are able to adjust to the changes that occur, and in doing so, embrace them. Even a so-called summer person can enjoy the change of elements that comes with winter. It becomes less about "bracing for winter" and more about experiencing the winter months for what they are. And even if winter drags into early spring, it matters less because the season will change. In fact, it already has, albeit subtly. We cannot master nature, but in mastering ourselves, we flow and adapt as the season changes in its own time.

Empowerment comes from recognizing the pluralism in everything and not fighting it. This also applies to the most common and yet unspoken pluralism: living and dying. The two are related and, as shown earlier, fall under Yang—events beyond our control. So why fight it? And why be afraid?

If our nature inspires thoughts that lead to actions that create results, why not focus your attention there? There is always a cause and an effect—living and dying is cause and effect, but what exists between those entities is action. Our actions. The cause initiates our response, which through action creates a result, or effect. The cycle continues in small and large exchanges in every moment of our life. In Pushing Hands we practice learning to receive the attack—the protagonist energy or cause—and then using that energy in a response that literally changes the outcome of the exchange. We are an active participant in the resulting effect. This is T'ai Chi's lesson in the art of living.

In Japan, the Samurai could not fight to their ultimate potential if they feared losing their lives in battle. Through practice, they would eventually release concern about killing or being killed and focus only on the actions of the enemy. The Samurai were able to respond without this additional layer of thought, which only slowed their reaction and increased the danger of defeat and death. By practicing an understanding of the natural cycles of life and death and training to act without fear, you become empowered to focus on the act. The lesson here is that life's battle will have already been fought in your training.

Then, maybe when you reach your final day and draw your last breath, it will be the result of a life lived in a way that was honest, engaged, and without fear. This is where your quality of life exists. And that quality of life will touch those around you in subtle or profound ways.

You change the world you live in by making a statement on how to live life well. This is your real legacy.

One of the primary roots of total wellness exists in living well: developing a sense of quality in our personal nature that endures over time and through endless cycles of change. The improved outlook influences state of mind, which transmits to the physical being. The root theory of T'ai Chi, that a healthy mind is critical for health and longevity, is certainly true. And you can start down the path to a healthy mind by acquiring an understanding, a perspective, and a way to interact with the natural world as each moment reveals itself in small or grand events.

Inspiration for Practice

BE THE STUDENT AND BE THE TEACHER. Your teachers provide a method and guidance to attain external knowledge through T'ai Chi's physical movement and discussion of its philosophy and intentions. But it is your job to conduct the inward focus. This is when you become your own teacher.

HOW DID
YOU SEE THAT?

Heightened Awareness

I was at a county fair, held annually on the campus of a local community college. My girlfriend and I were out for a double date with her sister and her sister's boyfriend, John. The four of us walked the perimeter, stopping to "whack a mole" or spend $15 to toss basketballs into misshapen hoops for a $2 stuffed animal prize. Harmless fun as the sun was beginning to set on a Long Island summer day.

The grounds were crowded with families, teenagers hanging out with friends, and twenty-somethings on dates. I have never been comfortable in crowds, so I tend to be quiet. John, however, talked. And talked. And talked. A lot. I wasn't sure if he felt the need to fill the silence or just to express every passing thought.

At one point the girls wanted an ice cream cone, so we stood near a tent as the girls ate and John continued his commentary. I became uncomfortable.

"I think it's time to go."

My girlfriend assumed that I'd become annoyed with John's nonstop talking. Which was true, but not the cause of my discomfort. I could feel that something was brewing.

I perceived a change in the environment, like a storm was gathering, gaining energy like a tornado. I looked at the crowd thirty feet away. What had been a relaxed rhythm of walking, strolling, or playing carnival games became fast and frenetic. People were moving to one side or another, like the parting of a sea.

Out from the crowd emerged two men, about nineteen or twenty years old, in a fierce battle. They swung violently to the left and right, punching, grabbing, and tugging until both came crashing down on a baby stroller. The parents looked down on the two young men with horror and anger. Luckily, the child was in her mother's arms.

There were no security guards, only bystanders, to break up the fight.

Fights between boys happen. It is a primordial seed that prepares them to be men. I'm not advocating violence but do recognize the fact. One must learn to fight for survival. One must also learn to focus and control the impulse when the "fight or flight" instinct is activated. And while someone can argue that we're less threatened in the modern world by a T. rex or tiger, a casual glance at the news will reveal that ordinary people are assaulted and attacked every day. But that was not the discussion after this fight.

"How did you see that?" my companions asked me.

I didn't know. I could just sense it somehow.

This sensation I experienced occurred ten years before I began to study martial arts, so it was undefined and unrefined. I did not understand it, nor could I explain it to someone. This was something I just sensed. Looking back, I always had sensed changes in the environment or in the energy of a room.

Sensing was a quality I always possessed but considered to be more of a condition. I was a sensitive kid in school. And being a sensitive kid, at least in Western culture, goes against the social norm. Someone like me who has an empathetic nature can become insecure, which I was. It was confusing to me.

I could perceive a slight change in someone's body language. A look from the corner of the eye, a tightening of the lip, someone turning their back; it was all absorbed and processed, but my lack of experience or knowledge made it difficult to understand and respond. Most of the time I was just unsure. It took almost thirty-five years to figure out that what I naturally possessed was not a weakness, but a strength.

Sensitivity is a characteristic of the world's introverts, and a strength among practitioners of T'ai Chi. But these characteristics are perceived inequitably within cultures that gravitate toward the big personality, the loud voice, or the large physique. There is a lack of recognition for the value offered by introverts—and T'ai Chi people, for that matter—even though they live in the same towns, work, raise families, spend money, vote, and are significant contributors to innovations in thinking, technology, philosophy, and business practice. Discounting their value limits the opportunity to leverage these complementary traits to elevate a society locally, regionally, or nationally.

We are all a combination of introversion and extroversion. The difference lies in one trait dominating our mode of relating to the world around us. Introverted people respond to a level of stimulation or an event sooner than an extrovert. Introverts seem to possess a heightened level of perception. People have a higher level of perception when they possess a peaceful mind and quiet temperament. This disposition is often overlooked in the West but traditionally respected in Eastern cultures. There, these people are not labeled as introverts. In a conversation this person will listen more than speak. When they do speak, people who recognize the value listen closely. Internally oriented people are respected and have influence. It is within this culture that an art like T'ai Chi can develop, be refined, and endure over centuries.

People who train as internal martial artists, known as T'ai Chi Chuan *adepts*, succeed in confrontation by developing their skills of "listening," or sensing. They use touch as a way of gathering and processing information. When it is performed with a clear or empty mind, the channels of communication between the mind and body are open and the interaction is instantaneous. With this skill, an internal martial artist possessing a heightened perception of the opponent's direction and level of force will respond sooner and more accurately.

T'ai Chi adepts do not display their intention or telegraph their strike. They use touch and sensitivity to read the opponent's intention and then ensnare their attack, forcing a committed position that ultimately works against the attacker. The internal martial artist—the introvert—changes the outcome. They respond to the encounter with greater power and less effort.

The pathway to this skill is developed and enhanced through constant practice of T'ai Chi Chuan. (T'ai Chi translates to "grand ultimate" and T'ai Chi Chuan to "grand ultimate fist.") A person with a more introverted personality will be drawn to the art, as many introverts employ a more deliberate process by their very nature. They understand and embrace a more nuanced course, trusting the results to come over time.

The person possessing a highly developed internal approach to the world lacks ego but is confident. They respond rather than initiate, but the response is assertive. Where others appear loud, edgy, pushy, or stressed beyond capacity, the internal person seems quiet and moves things along in a calm, almost effortless way. The effort may be so subtle that no one seems to notice because there is an absence of drama or fanfare; they just get things done.

The Master acts without doing anything.
And teaches without saying anything
Things arise and she lets them come

Things disappear and she lets them go
She has but doesn't possess
Acts but doesn't expect
When her work is done, she forgets it
That's why it lasts forever.

—*Tao de Ching*, Verse 2

Developing sensitivity and heightened awareness as a strength is no small feat, and isn't accomplished merely because one is naturally introverted and sensitive. A person possessing a highly skillful internal method has first recognized their nature and then sought instruction to develop the approach. They recognize and develop an area of strength.

You can find sources of insight and information in books like Susan Cain's *Quiet*, the writings of Gandhi, the *Tao de Ching*, and its practice through T'ai Chi. Like introverts themselves, however, these resources fly under the radar and compete for space among shelves of self-help books written by high-energy motivational authors, or among movies depicting aggressive action to gain results and sports favoring brute force over strategy.

This is not to say that introverted and thoughtful people have never occupied a place in America. A poem called "Desiderata" by Max Ehrmann contains wisdom and sage advice that relates equally to the *I Ching*, the Bible, and the writings of Rumi. Among these writings include:

- Go placidly among the noise and hassle and remember what peace there may be in silence.

- Speak your truth quietly and clearly; and listen to others . . . .

- Avoid loud and aggressive persons; they are vexatious to the spirit.

- Nurture strength of spirit to shield you in sudden misfortune.

- You are a child of the universe, no less than the trees and the stars; you have a right to be here.

- Whether or not it is clear to you, the universe is unfolding as it should.

- Whatever your labors and aspirations, in the noisy confusion of life, keep peace with your soul.

Language, metaphors, and allegories may differ, but since the beginning of humankind, all religions and philosophies have sought to express these universal truths. But these writings cannot fully describe something alive and moving, which makes it beyond fixed definitions and descriptions. T'ai Chi animates these truths beyond documents because the art is alive through its movement.

Universal truth exists in all parts of nature. It can be accessed when we silence ourselves through physical practice to discover the truth within ourselves. A person practicing T'ai Chi experiences a momentary glimpse into the principles expressed in the *Tao de Ching*: the nature of the universe. It is not a purely intellectual process, but rather a gateway to intelligence. With this newfound awareness you begin to perceive any deviation or nontruth, no matter how subtle. You acquire a heightened awareness. It is a soft power. And it is addicting.

In her book *Quiet,* Susan Cain devotes a chapter to soft power. She describes her pursuit of a class with a communication professor named Preston Ni. Ni acknowledges the need for a certain level of charismatic energy for brilliant people to have a voice in the US business culture. But he doesn't necessarily believe that the approach is superior. He presents the concept of soft power as a form of leading "by water rather than by fire," a more subtle but determined and skillful approach. He goes on to say, "Aggressive power beats you up, soft power wins you over." By acquiring greater awareness, you are better able to influence.

Applying this soft and subtle approach brings forth an awareness of how patterns unfold naturally. You align with the pattern, rather than fight it. You may let it carry you forward, even when you're unsure of the destination. You may let others pass. You also may help others pass by harnessing the natural pattern to influence their movement.

Open-mindedness, sensitivity, and a deep understanding of nature become potent tools for identifying and responding to these patterns of nature, the shifting currents of life. The T'ai Chi person will adjust, Yin or Yang, to the situation in order to create a balance. This dynamic is encoded in all the natural elements, including water.

In *The Secret Knowledge of Water,* Craig Childs describes a study by Colorado State University researcher Ellen

Wohl. Seeking to understand the channeled carvings of eroding bedrock in canyons, Wohl constructed a twelve-foot trough that could run up to six gallons of water per second at different angles. When the angle of the incline increased, the running water began to change its erosion pattern. As the gradient increased, the water created increasingly complex patterns to stabilize itself by dissipating excess energy.

"Be like water," Bruce Lee famously said. And since we are composed of approximately 60 percent water, it makes sense. If you accept that we not only are connected but in fact are part of nature itself, then perhaps you can take a step further to consider the possibility that the water within us moves with a purpose and so may influence our behaviors. Quite a leap, I know, but maybe taking Bruce's advice is not such a distant notion, after all.

Of course, water is not the only natural element that exists within us. In fact, everything on this planet is composed of some combination of the ninety-two naturally occurring elements. So, it's not quite accurate to say that we are connected to nature. We *are* nature. T'ai Chi is built on a philosophy that strives to understand and align with the naturally existing patterns.

The practice of T'ai Chi creates a physical alignment with these common natural elements, which operate in the universal patterns of nature. Through study and practice, we increase our awareness of the changes, movement, and deviation of these natural patterns, and thus are less influenced by anything else, including media representations, status, or material reward.

The Tao is called the Great Mother
Empty yet inexhaustible
It gives birth to infinite worlds
It is always present within you
You can use it any way you want.

—*Tao de Ching*, Verse 6

Nature is an endless combination and repetition of a very few laws. She hums the well-known air through innumerable variations.

—RALPH WALDO EMERSON

The *Tao de Ching* advocates aligning with nature, and that includes understanding and aligning with your own nature. Know yourself and how you naturally respond to interactions, circumstances, events, and conflict. In this sense, conflict is not limited to physical interaction; it could just as easily be unwelcome change.

We are nature and within us exists our human nature. Understanding human nature increases through study, meditation, and practicing the shapes that make up T'ai Chi forms. Daily practice improves insight and awareness by allowing our minds to "be empty" enough to spontaneously interact. False perceptions are minimized or removed. We become more adept at anticipating situations before they grow into larger events because we are aware of the unfolding conditions sooner. Ideally, we can identify and capitalize on opportunities, delays, or leverage points sooner than the opposing force. It is the reason we practice.

Awareness as Strategy

While on vacation in Mexico, I went to the beach early to practice. A couple passed, and I could see the man waving his fingers around, mocking me as some sort of New Age magician. His partner chuckled. I was not offended.

I realize that people won't be intimidated or challenged by someone practicing T'ai Chi because it contains no blatantly offensive movements. Each position is defensive as the starting point. Observe an adept playing a T'ai Chi form, and you will see the flowing movement. Look a little more closely for the roll of the wrist or knee. The T'ai Chi person will change direction. It seems gentle, unassuming, even harmless, so the easy assumption is that nothing is really going on.

The strategy of T'ai Chi is to envelop an offensive tactic with a corresponding defense, turning the offensive strike around and using the opponent's energy against them. It takes time and self-trust to make this form of self-defense effective, but those who master the approach tend to master more than just the art. They master themselves and become more masterful with situations as they arise at home, work, or on the street.

Yielding and redirecting attacks is an equally effective strategy for verbal conflicts. Most often a quiet approach that anticipates, yields, and then redirects the verbal attack will enable you to minimize politics and negativity; it's better to focus on what you are there to do. When this occurs, most people around you, distracted by the noise of their own desires, agenda, and insecurities, will never recognize that you did anything at all.

In this sense, T'ai Chi is a gateway to developing sensitivity into heightened awareness and prevention. Once you learn the T'ai Chi form, the inward focus becomes an instrument to achieve a better understanding of yourself. The mind and body increasingly function in concert with themselves. Over time, as this self-knowledge deepens, the physical body becomes more sensitive to change. It may be a change in environment, like temperature, or a change in the temperament of a crowd, as I unknowingly found out all those years ago at the county fair.

Everyday practice is a passageway to greater self-knowledge. That knowledge increases confidence and self-trust. Over time these qualities allow you to become less introverted, enabling you to see the bigger picture and engage with the outer world, communicating at a level beyond words: feeling, hearing, smelling, seeing, even tasting with an awareness as if it were the first time. You become less self-conscious. Your actions emanate from intention. You objectively observe and adjust to align and harmonize from your own place in the world. This is connecting to, and truly living within, the source and flow of life.

Think about a time when you took a trip to a different part of the country or the world. You can most likely recall the local accent and dress of the people you met. You remember the architecture of the buildings, or the topography of rivers, mountains, hills, and valleys. The streets may have been dirt, cobblestone, or pavement.

The weather was warmer, colder, drier, or more humid than you are accustomed to. The trees may have been different, as were the birds and type of pets you see. You remember the experience in detail because it was unique. But the ability to experience something in this way is not unique at all.

You can achieve this level of elation without spending $10,000 or $20,000 on an exotic vacation. You can experience newness and wonder right where you live. Try walking through your neighborhood or walk to work, but pretend you just arrived at a place you've never been before. You may recapture the excitement you felt when you first moved into your neighborhood, made a new friend, or started a new job.

For years I have counseled professionals on their career. The client may be a junior person trying to map a career path or late-stage professionals dealing with a change of circumstance and in need of career alternatives. During the sessions I ask them to conduct an exercise, and I will share the first part here.

With a pad of paper or a memo app on your phone or tablet, set out for a walk. It could be your neighborhood or anywhere you'd like. As you walk, look around and record the things you observe. Keep it simple. It could look like:

- Tree without leaves
- Dog
- Blue Dodge Charger
- Wind on the back of my neck

Let the list sit for a day before reviewing it. Then, ask yourself: How new are these things? Have I noticed them before? In the next phase of the exercise these elements are put to work, but hopefully this simple first step has illustrated how you can heighten your awareness in places that are already familiar. You become more present. A walk in the neighborhood can become your meditation. It is simple but requires some discipline.

For example, want to increase awareness of all the things in your kitchen? Practice the T'ai Chi sword or saber form in that room without hitting anything. You'll become aware through touch or sound (hitting the refrigerator or knocking something over, as I have) of what exactly is around you. Your sphere of awareness grows larger.

Practicing T'ai Chi brings you to a state of presence in the flow of life, with the same awareness of the exotic journey. You regain a sense of newness, or renewal, every day. Each morning is experienced as a new event. Through practice you treat each inhale and exhale as unique. Every step is taken with mindfulness. You trace the motion of your arms and hands to better smooth the lines and arcs. Through this process you re-create yourself and, in that re-creation, have an opportunity to create your path of life. This is the secret, the fountain of youth.

Cultivating a present mind, which enables heightened awareness, through the discipline of T'ai Chi will inform and enhance other pursuits in your life. As our mind and body relax more deeply, our sphere of perception increases and widens. We become more aware of our surroundings. Our sense of awareness is heightened during travel because everything we see, touch, hear, and smell is new. We want to experience this new thing to the fullest. Whether far away or close to home, we develop the same view of the world by practicing awareness every day. The life cultivated through T'ai Chi is a living meditation of interacting, conversing, or exchanging as each moment is revealed, like music unfolding during a performance by master musicians.

In his introduction to jazz drummer Peter Erskine's autobiography *No Beethoven*, Mitch Haupers describes and praises Peter's approach to the instrument, encapsulating a lifetime of disciplined self-improvement and success into three rules, which I believe can also be applied to T'ai Chi:

MASSIVE PREPARATION. This is akin to studying and developing your T'ai Chi to the fullest, including understanding the philosophical basis of the art, practicing Qi Gong and forms, and learning and applying self-defense applications like Pushing Hands and weapons.

NO EGO. Because Peter has practiced his drumming, and the music he has composed or is asked to record or perform for someone else, he can move his ego aside. This means that there is less need to monitor, evaluate, decide, and maybe even change all the things that interrupt and distract you from the very thing you endeavor to do.

If you are presenting or practicing a T'ai Chi form in public or are engaged in a Pushing Hands exchange, any presence of the ego will occupy part of your attention, which robs the venture of your full concentration. Reducing or removing the ego from the equation elevates performance.

REALLY LISTEN. When high-level musicians perform, they are participating in a musical conversation among the band members and between the band and the audience. Musicians must make contributions that support or add to the conversation in an appropriate way. What is or is not appropriate is measured by how it relates to the core, or essence, of the music. Just like in any conversation, you must first listen before blurting out a point of view! The music tells the musician what to do, if they listen closely. Since T'ai Chi is built on a principle of interaction, you must listen, mainly through touch, to respond.

I am not aware that Peter Erskine has studied or practiced T'ai Chi, but his approach to drumming and music has been called Zen. It's easy to see why when you understand his focus. Sounds a lot like awareness to me.

* * *

We've been discussing how heightened awareness informs and enriches your evolving life, but it's also a critical element in life preservation, as a defense strategy. Developing sensitivity and awareness to a high level enhances the ability to identify emerging patterns in potentially dangerous situations, as I experienced in my earlier story about the county fair. The skill will enable you to better sense when trouble arises, be it an argument, a conflict, or an attack. You may not always be consciously aware, but hopefully you will have heard that voice inside you, the instinct that motivates action and response. The key is to be ahead of the event and avoid trouble whenever possible. And that possibility exists with heightened awareness.

Avoiding trouble should always be the first option. Regardless of skill level, intense conflict is unpredictable, chaotic, and dangerous. You have no control of the other person, don't know what they know, and can't predict how they will act. Even the best-trained person can be taken by surprise or attacked in their blind spot. If you sense trouble, the first and best thing to do is walk across the street, walk the other way, or even run if you must.

If you can't avoid a face-to-face conflict, then the next option is to attempt to talk it out. This doesn't mean to surrender or let down your guard; you're attempting to control or contain the situation with diplomacy. Because just as you don't want to be hurt, you probably wouldn't want to harm another person unless you really must. It might come to that.

In an intense conflict you may run out of time or options. If at this point, there is a genuine concern for your life, your last and only course of action may be to physically defend yourself. And if that is an option that you decide to pursue, then it must be wholehearted. You must be committed. Your preparation, practice of no ego (you absolutely don't want to be monitoring yourself right now), and concentration will be drawn upon in real time and with serious consequences. Awareness is critical. A mistake or misstep can be costly.

T'ai Chi fighting skills center on mid-range and close-range fighting, so the listening skills described earlier enhance your overall fighting technique. Practicing Pushing Hands drills develops a higher sense of touch. Being able to sense changes in pressure or force from your opponent will give you a timely advantage. While your opponent has committed their force and speed in a direction, you remain soft and yielding and can use your higher level of awareness to perceive the speed, direction, and force level to respond earlier.

Having the ability to perceive an incoming force and knowing what to do next are different things. A person with the highest level of sensitivity may feel the force coming at them, but not know what to do about it. Instead, they allow the force to move forward, which traps and collapses the defense. At the extreme opposite, sensitivity and awareness has a maximum level of effectiveness and won't work against overwhelming force. You also practice T'ai Chi's martial applications to develop the appropriate responses.

Through practice, trial, and error, a T'ai Chi practitioner will become more aware of the variables they face along with options to defend, counter, and attack, or, in

T'ai Chi terms, *yield, redirect,* and *issue*—the root of the art's fighting philosophy. Practicing the forms improves coordination, proper breathing, relaxation, and body alignment for increased power. Pushing Hands and related drills heighten sensitivity and the ability to thwart attacks. Trapping drills and sparring increase the intensity and unpredictability of confrontation. When combined, these drills and exercises simulate scenarios that will sharpen your awareness and response with control and accuracy during violent conflict.

It is worth noting that in each training scenario, practitioners will make mistakes and hopefully learn a lesson for the next encounter. Heightened awareness takes on a different meaning here because we come to recognize patterns of attack and effective counteractions with techniques expressing their own path of force. It is only through experience and mistakes that lessons are learned, and in a contact-based art, it can bruise the body or the ego—or sometimes both.

Whether you're a natural introvert or not, pursuing and developing your inner nature through the practice of an internal art like T'ai Chi has many benefits. Clearing the mind creates relaxed awareness. Relaxed awareness increases perception. When these are developed through the art, you learn a rare skill and are more empowered. You are able to fully connect with your environment, to live in the moment, and to recognize clues or symptoms of change early enough to respond in a way that nurtures or protects your way of life.

Inspiration for Practice

VISUALIZE YOURSELF. Sometimes when I can't sleep or I'm waiting in a doctor's office or airport, I use the time to practice mentally. I picture myself going through the form. I am paying attention to each movement and seeking to crystallize my ideal vision of the perfect form. Visualization changes brain waves and evokes muscular change. It is the most powerful resource.

WISDOM AND FIGHTING SPIRIT IN THE FACE OF HOSTILITY

The martial arts originally evolved as a system to defend against thieves or invasions. The training included Qi Gong systems to calm the mind and control the emotions of the warrior. The foundational theory divides the mind into wisdom (Yi) and emotion (Xin). The earliest form of Qi Gong, one of the three roots of T'ai Chi, focused on regulating the mind, as it was believed that a healthy mind was essential for total well-being. Regulating the mind would eventually enable the practitioner to regulate their Qi, but it was and still is intended to bring the practitioner's mind into a deep and profound state of relaxation. It is from this state of being that we are able to recognize a growing or existing offensive and respond spontaneously, as opposed to reacting impulsively.

Qi Gong sets and T'ai Chi Chuan are built on the foundation of a still mind as regulated through breathing practices and meditation. Breathing patterns have a direct link to, and impact on, our emotional state. An angry person will use short, fast breaths, and a sad person will inhale more than exhale, for example. Because the mind is related to and directs the Qi, the emotional state of mind will have a direct impact on physical health and overall spirit. Through constant practice we learn to neutralize and redirect or remove thoughts that are illusory or negative. We increase our focus, concentration, and ability to experience and respond to events, problems, or conflicts without internalizing the encounter and risking trauma. Less emotion, more objectivity. More detachment, less stress.

Qi Gong theory divides the Qi into two categories: Fire Qi and Water Qi. Fire Qi is generated from food and air and is linked to one's emotions. Water Qi, or Original Qi, is rooted in Original Jing: the existing Qi in the body. This originates in the kidneys and is associated with wisdom. The goal of Qi Gong practice is to balance Fire and Water to control the emotional state and the physical condition, which impacts your Shen (spirit, soul, or higher being).

Shen exists in the elevated state when it is harmonized by the Yi or wisdom mind (Water Qi) and Xin or emotional mind (Fire Qi). A person living in this state is inspired and has clarity and greater sensitivity to change. When the Shen is raised by emotion, it must also be regulated by the Yi. Yi, Xin, and Shen are interconnected, and each is impacted and regulated by the other two. We exist at the highest potential state when the three are balanced.

By observing someone's behavior, you may gather clues about the relationship of their Xin, Yi, and Shen. Observe their actions and interactions with people. Who is going to great lengths to explain themselves? Who sighs every time they're asked to do something? Who is having an emotional outburst over poor service? Who seeks to control others in the group? Who seems relaxed and calm? Who is responsive? Who listens when another speaks?

With awareness and a little practice, you may find yourself recognizing the dominant Qi—Water or Fire—and adjusting your response in a way that balances your interaction with that person. This alone can significantly alter the results during a confrontation. We can manage the outcome, as opposed to allowing ourselves to be caught in someone else's domain, a seed of conflict, and then reacting in our own unfocused or uncontrollable way.

* * *

We stood on the platform with our guests, waiting for the train that would take us to Manhattan for some sightseeing. It was a pleasant summer day, and our friends were excited about what we had planned. I was up for it, too, but had noticed a lone man, perhaps homeless, orbiting closer to our group. This is a highly unusual thing for this area of Long Island, but my friends noticed nothing and continued to chirp on about what they wanted to see in Manhattan: the Ed Sullivan Theater, the Statue of Liberty, *any* New York pizza. The stranger moved closer and now stood face-to-face with my wife.

"That's a nice necklace. Can I have it?"

Silence.

My wife and friends were shocked at how brazen this person was. And I would have been, too, but my reaction was different than when I was younger. Back then, if I were confronted by a bully at school, I would feel the tension rise and only when it reached a breaking point would I be moved to action. My thinking then was tight and frantic, confused, and emotional. I would lash out at the opponent, sometimes successful, other times not. I was not in control of my situation. Instead, the situation controlled my thoughts and actions. But this day was different, and after years of training I've come to know why.

When this event took place, I'd been studying kung fu and T'ai Chi for a few years, but up until this time I'd never had an occasion to apply that training. In this situation, instead of looking at the man and letting my emotions build to an explosion, I looked at him and my mind began, in an ordered and lucid way, to race through an endless stream of responses and strategies that were developed over years of training. If this person were to grab with the right hand, I had a response. If he stepped forward with the left leg, I had another response, and so on. This mentality gave me peace of mind and, with that, I could look the stranger in the eye and tell him to move on.

When I did, the man hesitated. He looked at me to assess my level of fear. Was I bluffing or committed to action? He could tell that I wasn't intimidated. He calculated the odds. Maybe I knew something that he did not. The man retreated and moved on. My friends were impressed and wanted to brag about it on the train. I did not—*not at all.* I just wanted to call my Sifu to thank him. He was the one who taught me to fight without fighting.

Rivalry triggers our natural fight or flight response, but that response can be moderated by the breathing techniques that thread the Qi Gong and T'ai Chi systems. The intention is to control the response in our nervous system—to regulate the level of emotion, the corresponding biochemistry, and their combined impact on our frame of mind. We focus on developing the parasympathetic nervous system, which slows the process down by reducing our blood pressure and heart rate, which increase and intensify when the sympathetic nervous system is activated. These Qi Gong systems condition us for hostile encounters and enable us to gauge dimensions of battle spontaneously and unconsciously, calmly and objectively.

We learn and practice how to regulate Qi Gong as part of our T'ai Chi training, which creates a stable condition to work from, and maintains it as levels of engagement increase in our Pushing Hands, self-defense, and sparring drills. As noted previously, T'ai Chi's martial style (T'ai Chi Chuan) is centered on mid-range and close-range fighting. You learn to close the gap on your opponent and vary your technique to adapt or gain an advantage during the fight. These training drills teach how T'ai Chi's self-defense applications realistically work with an opponent.

The softness, or fluidity, of T'ai Chi is one of its defining characteristics within the martial arts family of styles. The technique is highly effective because it is disarming; the opponent rarely detects a pending threat. It also enables you to use touch to follow the opponent's action so that you can find openings and opportunities to strike.

You'll need to learn how to best apply the self-defense strategies within an area of space. How much area is available for movement? Observing the environment of the engagement will inform how you decide to position yourself. When I encountered that man at the train station, I needed to assess the distance between us and the edge of the platform. I needed to mitigate the risk of us falling to the ground, wrestling, and rolling onto the track with a train due to arrive at any moment. Know your arena.

T'ai Chi practitioners who spend time on Pushing Hands drills and sparring gain valuable knowledge in how to apply their strategies and, just as importantly, learn how to time their technique. This is a dimension of action that is largely missed by people in an elevated emotional state who are driven by impulse; they react without thinking. They lose their rhythm, so their poorly timed responses work against them.

Sticking, adhering, neutralizing, and redirecting are the cornerstones of T'ai Chi's martial arts techniques, but you must know the right moment to apply them. The application of these techniques, along with your counter-attacks, may occur in the late stage of your confrontation. You may initially need to focus on blocking and avoiding an opponent who attacks in an uncontrolled and unpredictable way. It is critical to remain calm, observant, agile, and ready. There isn't time to "think." You must truly flow.

Most people don't understand how T'ai Chi is used in a martial way. They don't realize that there's more than one method and option for combating opponents. For instance, the legendary T'ai Chi elder Yang Ch'eng Fu advised responding to brute force with cleverness and to cleverness with power. We may address high postures with low or apply circular fighting techniques against linear fighting techniques, for example. The options are endless if your fundamentals are strong. Each dimension of this fighting style takes time to learn, develop, and integrate into your arsenal. You practice until your body can move on its own. You develop an agile and adaptive mind.

You also must know, or quickly learn, the opponent. Some of this is the result of practice, but it also must happen as the event unfolds in real time. Our ability to recognize, synthesize, and respond to stimuli in the ideal mental, emotional, and physical state empowers the intellect to respond and direct intention efficiently in real time, as the engagement develops. Clear, open-minded intelligence enables us to gather real-time information and then respond spontaneously and appropriately, without the interference of the conscious thinking that labels, evaluates, measures, and envisions possible outcomes—each of which contributes a layer of stress that has no direct relationship to the actual conflict. Quieting, reducing, and eventually eliminating this stress-inducing conscious thinking is one of the greatest rewards for dedicated T'ai Chi practice.

There are martial arts stories about renowned figures possessing incredible skills and legendary abilities to instantly respond to surprise situations. These stories, sometimes bordering on mythical, most often describe how a T'ai Chi master was able to sense and interpret body language and a minor change in condition. They read the intention early and had a timely response. Their mind was present.

There is a link to present mind and spirit. That link is courage. Courage is a mental and moral quality that animates your actions. It is stepping off the ledge into the unknown with a willingness to fail, or to be hurt, or to lose—whether that means losing an opportunity, a possession, a relationship, a fight, or a life as you once knew it. There are no guarantees, even for the best trained. Courage acknowledges the potential loss, even if briefly, but compels movement nonetheless.

Courage and confidence can be developed through consistent training and testing in the martial form of T'ai Chi Chuan. With the right teacher, you can step into it slowly and at your own pace. Still, this isn't easy for many people to do. Most people don't seek T'ai Chi training to fight. We each train for our own reasons, and I'm guessing that you're not seeking to fight. I don't want to fight either, but I do want to be prepared. To have peace of mind.

You need courage and confidence to enter the ring of hostility, because it's going to get ugly in there. But remember that courage, confidence, and spirit without wisdom can just as easily lead to defeat. Entering a battle that you know you'll lose when you have an opportunity to walk or run away isn't courageous—it's stupid. Have the wisdom to be intelligent and understand your purpose.

You must have the right purpose for your actions. There must be a reason to win. You must be committed to every act. We see this exemplified in stories about the underdog who overcomes seemingly insurmountable odds for a victory. They have a cause. You must have a purpose.

The resolution of the fight is also dependent on your own moral compass. If you seek to do harm as retribution, then you're not acting correctly. You will cause ancillary damage physically, morally, professionally, or reputationally. There is always a consequence. Your response leaves a trail.

Can you lose a confrontation and still have peace of mind? Yes, if your purpose was right and you were committed to your actions. There is a greatness in that, regardless of outcome. And if you consider the alternative, then also consider that avoidance of a hostility still has an effect on you.

Confrontation is generally something that people would rather avoid. Some feel challenged, while others feel bullied. Emotions begin to run in a negative direction and people become uncomfortable. Depending on the level of perceived friendliness and competence, attitudes toward the other person can range from distrust, envy, contempt, anger, or injustice to vulnerability and helplessness. These emotions are intense and have a direct impact on our physical well-being.

When I dealt with the pain of confrontation in the past, some of my responses were harsh, angry, or negative (I'm a master of sarcasm), which did more harm than good. Training in T'ai Chi changed that. It exposed me to a practical strategy to balance the wisdom and emotional dimensions of myself. This balance strengthened my spirit. It helped me face the hostilities of the day without triggering the fight or flight pattern. Instead, I could receive and respond to frictions, collisions, contrasts, conflicts, and attacks regardless of the intensity. These exchanges have an energy that we can use to amplify our own power.

You and the object of your inquiry are dependent upon each other.

> *Working together, the interaction of your spheres of influence can achieve significant deeds. Synergistic interaction will provide surplus energy for continued growth.*

> —*I Ching*, Chapter 30

* * *

Think about a time when you were in a public space that had potential for a fight to break out, like a local dive bar. With some awareness, many times you could see the signals long before the actual fight. Look around the next time you're in such a place. You may recognize it in the expression on someone's face. You may sense the raised level of Qi as the person walks past. Watch further to see how they interact with the people around them, including their response and level of animated gestures.

You may be in a situation like this and thinking, *How will I know what to do?* This is the right question to ask. What would you do? I ask that question every time a situation like this presents itself, and to be honest, some days I think I have a clear answer and other days I don't. Which one is better?

I think it's the days that I don't know how I'd respond. Here's why: I'm not yet in the situation. I'm not in the situation because it hasn't yet occurred. Since it hasn't occurred, I don't yet have the information needed to inform a response.

A threatening-looking person acting out twenty feet away from you is not yet a threat. They may not even be concerned about you. But if that person approaches you, then your mind will begin to make quick assessments. By remaining calm and keeping your head clear, you'll make minor observations. Is this person's center of gravity high? Are they leading with the right or left hand? Are they winding up to punch? The brain of a trained practitioner will generate a response that is as effective as one can be.

You have a strategic and tactical advantage if you've identified this person as a potential problem from the outset, and this is a critical component of entering a fight with success. Training in T'ai Chi develops a mindset to see the macro picture, to remain calm, and to let the body and mind function without the interference of conscious thought or ego.

The assailant draws nearer. You feel the rush of adrenaline. Your heart beats faster. Blood streams through your veins. Many people label this as nervousness or fear. In reality, the Yi—the wisdom mind—has activated your system and is readying the body for the encounter. Emotion and spirit are raised but *focused*. It is at this point when the flight or fight reaction discussed earlier is actually *supposed* to happen. Do you see the difference?

We train to be relaxed the majority of the time so that when we enter this heightened mental, physical, and spiritual level, it's only for a short period of time and for the appropriate action. Don't resist the sensation when it occurs, even if it feels like nervous excitement. Don't let the ego creep in to review and question every move you make. Daily T'ai Chi practice is intended to train the student to allow this process without becoming overwhelmed by it. It is more like an expansion of energy—an awakening. The Qi becomes an energy field. The energy animates martial movement through the engagement with your opponent. It can be exhilarating, and a little startling, when you experience the sensation. But it's a magnificent feeling. And it's most effective when you get out of your own way.

Inspiration for Practice

PRACTICE IN REAL TIME.   Be totally immersed in what you are doing at that particular moment. If you remove the "thinking," then your mind will relax and reveal the deeper self. Your inner world, in turn, is expressed in your movement as you practice the T'ai Chi form, perform Pushing Hands, or engage in self-defense. These expressions are your art, like playing a piece of music. When your inner world is in order, you can better respond to external conflict as the world spins around you.

THE CIVIL AND MARTIAL
SIDES OF T'AI CHI

"World peace" is the answer most associated with beauty pageant contestants. Maybe their response has become cliché because it's among our highest ideals. I'd also like to believe that most, if not all, people prefer to live life peacefully. Peace is a civil aspiration. It is what motivates us to let another person go first or to talk through a confrontational situation. It is at the heart of compromise and flexibility. Civility represents the "better angels of our nature," as President Abraham Lincoln said.

But here's the rub: life is never going to be that smooth. There will always be someone who wants more, someone who is angry, someone who is hurt, someone who seeks retribution or revenge. There will always be a collision of principles, philosophies, religion, cultures, and ways of life. There will always be discord. Sooner or later a conflict of some sort will knock on your door. When it does, you must choose a response. Essentially, you must decide to respond in a civil or martial way. This choice is ingrained into more areas of life than we can imagine, so understanding and mastering both options is important. This initial decision will drive the subsequent choices and actions we take while progressing through an encounter. This is not a new dynamic. It is an essential question that has been pondered and addressed for thousands of years.

The civil/martial choice has been part of our decision-making process since the beginning of tribes and the formation of early societies. It has been part of every treatise written about conflict or war. The first line of *The Art of War* states: "Conflict is essential to the development and growth of man and society." *The Art of War*'s principles and strategies follow the acknowledgment and acceptance of conflict as a fact of life. The document plans for war, but also for peace. Likewise, T'ai Chi's classical documents of principles and instruction recognize this fact. These ancient records teach students to understand the symbiosis: civil as the essence and martial as the function.

I never imagined that these statements could impact my perspective of life so profoundly, but they have. I am by nature more civil in disposition. My life focus has been on arts and humanities. Fighting was something that I actively avoided. I didn't like it. Still don't. But by learning the relationship and necessity of civil *and* martial approaches—a fighter's spirit—I became a more complete person. I was able to be myself without compromise. I could advocate for others. I could stand up against bullies. I could learn how to cultivate and preserve peace in a conflicted world. Here is what I learned.

* * *

According to the T'ai Chi classics, the civil side of the equation consists of inner principles, the ideals and values held personally and within a society. It is also the baseline of interaction between people, and as such it defines one's character, because to maintain civility during a conflict isn't always easy.

Most people are not aware of, do not understand, or have little education or training in civility. Many believe that we live in a civilized world and so civility simply exists, but in fact it is the result of centuries of evolution. In the modern world, for example, waiting patiently on an express check-out line when the person before you has clearly ignored the maximum item allowance is being civil. Choosing not to yell at a neighbor whose dog is barking late at night is being civil. These are easy examples. If we increase the impact of the encounter even slightly, we can see how civility begins to evaporate.

When my daughter was three years old, I took her to an Easter egg hunt sponsored by the village. They grouped the kids by age and spread the eggs across a large field so that every child could find a few eggs to enjoy. When the town official signaled the start of the hunt, I let my daughter wander out onto the field. I noticed then that she was being quickly passed by parents holding their children in their arms and running to gather as many eggs as they could hold. What started as an idealistic family day turned into a game of survival. Courtesy, patience, and awareness of the bigger picture gave way to "he who has the most, wins."

That is one isolated event. Now let's intensify the circumstance.

Perhaps the most accessible illustration of something that is civil, even beyond civil, is love. Love is truly a higher state of interaction, and yet it can invert to one of the nastiest, most bitter human interactions. That usually occurs at the breakup of an intense love affair or upon divorce. It is rare when a couple who were once in love, shared a home, and raised kids can end their marriage with civility. A relationship that was built around trust, cooperation, flexibility, giving, patience, and joy often descends into deceit, stubbornness, betrayal, anger, and a willingness to hurt the other emotionally, financially, and materially. Civility is replaced by an angry war, and the damage can be great.

Civility can exist on a sliding scale of sorts. It is a moving target. It is not always easy to maintain. In the extreme, what's sometimes labeled as civility may just be a lack of willingness to stand up for oneself or for what is morally right. Sometimes people trying to keep the peace are just being lazy. They don't want the disruption, so they allow themselves or someone else to be subjected to the impulsive or controlling action of another person. This idle obedience to civility often ends with an injured party. The passivity of the victim is at least partly liable here.

What if something occurred that demands a response that's not civil but martial? Would you see the martial response as evil? And are you prepared to respond in that way if required? Here's where the confusion lies: people often regard martial and civil as opposites, but they're not. The two are interconnected, a Yin and Yang, two sides of the same coin.

The divorcing spouse who justifies every nasty action isn't choosing the martial option over civility; they're simply abandoning their civility. And the other spouse, who accepts, internalizes, and becomes scarred by the actions of their ex, has neither the knowledge nor the nerves to summon a martial response. They don't fight for themselves, so they become a victim. One party ignored their inner principle; the other, an external technique.

Martial technique is a tool intended to complement your inner principle and preserve civility. The martial side of the equation isn't to be expressed from anger and can't be the sole personal doctrine of any person. Civility must still exist at one's core. Without it, the martial person is a brute or a thug—force without purpose.

* * *

I had a strange experience that turned out to be a lesson for me. I'd boarded a train after a long day. I sat down and settled in, then took a few minutes to massage some pressure points, a daily ritual that helps reduce tension in my body after I've worked for many hours. I try to be subtle, and most people don't even pay attention. But today someone was watching.

Across the aisle sat a man in his early thirties. His body was twisted into the corner of the seat, almost like a trapped animal. His leg was shaking. He would look at me with dull eyes. When I would notice and face him, his eyes would dart away. With so many news reports of soft target terrorist attacks, or ordinary citizens suddenly attacking people around them (during this writing there was an attack in a Manhattan hospital), I was concerned. Passengers sitting around us displayed body language that telegraphed their discomfort, too. They focused their attention on the movies and video games on their devices. Their choice was to bury their heads in the sand. Would you consider that a civil response?

Why is this guy so nervous? I asked myself. I looked over at the man and his belongings to determine if he had concealed anything. The moments unfolded, and I neared a decision point.

Instead of meditating with my eyes closed, I decided to remain aware of this person. I also decided to post the incident on social media. I'm not sure what motivated this. Maybe it was to document the occurrence in the event something really transpired. But not long after, as responses to the post began to mount, I realized that this was also an opportunity to learn about how someone might react if they were in my place.

The responses from friends and acquaintances included advice to leave the train car, confront the stranger, report him, ignore him, and be ready to fight. Split into two basic categories, the responses were basically fight or flight. I chose a response that was not recommended by anyone. I said hello.

The man responded. "Do you have a headache?"

"No," I said, "I'm trying to prevent one. I do this little self-massage routine each day to relax after working. It seems to help."

"Do you work in New York and then travel to Long Island every day?"

"Yes. You get used to it."

With that, the man went on to explain that he wasn't from here. I began to understand that his agitation was rooted in discomfort. He was lost and a little confused, and there seemed to be some mild form of mental illness involved. We kept talking.

After twenty minutes, he began to settle down. His body settled into the seat, he began to distract himself with his phone, and his leg stopped shaking. The surrounding passengers relaxed, too.

The entire encounter didn't last long and in hindsight seems harmless. But we live in an unpredictable time, so you never really know when an incident like this can escalate and become dangerous. The different social media opinions about how to address this situation included some correct options—that can't be overstated. My point is that when you have both civil and martial options, you're able to start with civility. You can start with civility because with martial skills you're less fearful. Less fearful means clear thinking. Clear thinking means not overacting.

My first choice was civility—but civility that could be followed by martial intent, if required. And, as I learned, a martial response is the last response. Then you must make it count.

In modern society we seem to have forgotten the need to balance the civil and martial behaviors within ourselves. Civil has become passivity. Martial has become violence. The polarity is evidenced in the attitude of citizens and actions of politicians who preach for peace while undermining mechanisms that maintain the law.

There have been news reports highlighting police brutality and wrongful deaths over the last couple of years. Some are clearly the wrongdoing of the police officer, but not all. In any such event, there must always be investigation and accountability. But if the reflex action is to reduce the martial efficacy of law enforcement, then we risk converting the function into a purely civil role, rendering the police ineffective in carrying out the duties of their job, and in some cases becoming victims themselves. This subject is deserving of analysis, debate, and potential solutions, which is beyond the scope of this book. But the circumstance is common to all of us, so it's instructive to view the role of a police officer within the context of civility and martial intent. One reported incident got me thinking.

The news reported a story about three police officers who, when attempting to arrest a very large man, forced him to the ground in a chokehold. The man said that he could not breathe and later died. For the sake of inquiry, let's put aside the criminal record of the alleged perpetrator and any record of abuse by one officer, if it exists. Through the prism of civil and martial options, the questions that emerged for me were: Why did the police officer feel compelled to use this level of force? Why was his takedown of the man so brutal? What options did the officer have? Why does the family blame the police or claim that the system failed them? Why does a mayor insist on additional sensitivity training knowing that this particular neighborhood has high crime and is dangerous?

A few days later I was at a family gathering attended by a cousin who is a police officer. It was a great opportunity to get some insight. I asked, "How many times a year are you required to visit the shooting range in order to hold your gun?"

The answer was twice a year.

"How often are you required to train in open-hand takedowns?"

And then I heard the answer I hoped I wouldn't: "We don't train in open-hand takedowns after basic training."

From this conversation I realized that we have a system that takes young and inexperienced men and women, provides them with a few weeks of training, and sends them into dangerous, high-crime areas with guns that, if used, will be held against them by media and politicians low on information but assuming a higher moral position. The system failed the police—and failed our citizens.

Sending an inexperienced and undertrained armed person into a dangerous area is like sending them into a war zone. They are constantly on guard and seek only to live through the day—to survive—so that they can go home. I'm willing to bet that most of these people are so tense and high-strung that when an event escalates and prompts a lethal response, they just cannot turn it off. The fight or flight trigger goes into full effect here, with potentially severe consequences for everyone involved.

What if our police were trained to be experts in civility *and* martial intent? It seems to me that the first mandate of a patrolling officer is to develop a rapport and relationship with the citizens they're there to protect. They should extend respect, but also be respected. An officer of the law shouldn't have to perform their job with trepidation about encounters with criminals and gang members. When enforcing the law and keeping the peace, police officers must be empowered and supported by proper training, the neighborhood, its citizens, politicians, and the media. The police must also responsibly carry out their sworn duty as people who enforce the law without being above it. Society thrives in a safe environment, which is achieved when there's a balance of principles and technique.

Our law enforcement system is designed to maintain civility by protecting our citizens. The role of a police officer isn't to be diminished. Instead, they should be well trained and required to continuously improve their level of martial skill while respecting and supporting the value of their code of conduct.

Martial force must exist. To deny its necessity is to naively hope for a life without conflict or pain. This simply does not, and won't ever, exist. But it's important to realize that the ultimate goal of any martial action is to facilitate a return to peace. This principle must be the gauge used for any aggressive action by a citizen, law enforcement officer, military general, or politician contemplating war. It is the essence of the martial arts.

Shaolin martial arts was not created with a violent intent, but rather to respond to external hostility. As David Chow and Richard Spangler write in *Kung Fu: History, Philosophy and Technique*, "Kung fu should be used only to preserve the natural flow of life, to avoid, divert, neutralize or blend with any destructive force." To only use martial skill for violence or murder would be to disgrace the art, its ideals, and its values.

When the monk Bodhidharma traveled from India to China, he brought exercise forms to unite and elevate the body and mind with perfection of the self as the goal. The heightened fitness of the body and mind was a gateway to deeper meditation with the goal of attaining enlightenment. The motivation for these exercises was rooted in civility as *spirituality*. It evolved into a martial art only in response to threats against the Shaolin monks' way of life.

The notion that monks in the Shaolin temple did nothing more than train to become elite fighters is false. They did train out of martial necessity, but that was not their exclusive focus. Monks also learned to master philosophy, writing and calligraphy, poetry, and music. These arts, when combined with martial training, became a whole that was greater than the sum of the parts. The individual process of self-cultivation through rigorous mental and physical rituals raised the spirit— the supreme goal. They cultivated civility through the martial arts training.

Author Alan Watts said, "Believing is clinging, faith is letting go." Many people amble through life believing that trouble will somehow pass them by. But should it arrive, they believe the trouble will be addressed by a higher authority: a parent, a police officer, a doctor, a benefactor, or the government. This person has not developed faith in themselves during periods of opposition or altercation. But self-faith is required because conflict is chaotic or unpredictable. Self-faith can be cultivated through martial training.

Learning martial morality from an art like T'ai Chi is a tremendous benefit. It is a portal to understanding life's hardships. It is through this understanding that your civil and martial philosophy will grow as a deep and genuine part of your humanity. You learn the interplay and balance between these two seemingly polar opposites that are eternally connected. Even though this process includes bumps and bruises to the body and ego, the results justify the means.

* * *

The iconic television show *M*A*S*H* included an episode titled "Heroes." For those who may never have watched the show, *MASH* is an acronym for Mobile Army Surgical Hospital. The unit was staffed with doctors and nurses during the Korean War. One of the main characters is Father Mulcahy, the unit's bewildered and forgiving chaplain.

In this episode Father Mulcahy's hero, prizefighter "Gentleman Joe" Cavanaugh, visits the *MASH* unit and, while there, suffers a stroke. At the bedside of the unconscious man, Father Mulcahy shares his own story, and why Cavanaugh is his hero. The scene eloquently and perfectly illustrates this chapter's theme.

Father Mulcahy tells of his life as a bookish child and explains that Plato was his first hero. Mulcahy loved Plato's notion that perfection isn't found in this imperfect world, but rather in some dimension or universe—an "ideal plane"—that can't be perceived by humans. This idealism made young Mulcahy a target for the neighborhood bullies. Fighting back went against the Platonic principles, so his childhood was a life of torment.

At twelve years old, Mulcahy witnessed his second hero, "Gentleman Joe" Cavanaugh, in the boxing ring. Cavanaugh dominated the match. The crowd worked up to a frenzy. They cheered and yelled at him to finish off the other man. Instead, Cavanaugh stepped back. He told the referee to end the match. His opponent had been beaten. There was no need to hurt him more.

The experience was a turning point for Father Mulcahy: "That was when I made up my mind to keep one foot in the ideal plane and the other foot in the real world."

Practice the civil and the martial. This is self-cultivation.

Inspiration for Practice

HOW YOU PRACTICE IS HOW YOU PERFORM. Your T'ai Chi form, Pushing Hands, and self-defense drills must be practiced with intention. Even if you are not hitting your training partner with full force, your mind must be focused on the strike. This is because the mind directs your energy in the area where you are focused. It is what animates your technique with impactful power. When you practice with a sense of enemy, you are training a real response for when you need it.

INNER STRENGTH
AND VIRTUE

Express yourself completely
Then keep quiet,
Be like the force of nature
When it blows, there is only wind
When it rains, there is only rain
When the clouds pass, the sun shines through.

—*Tao de Ching*, Verse 23

The *Tao de Ching* is a timeless treasure. It endures because it communicates grand principles to contemplate and apply in your own life. This verse taught me to trust my nature.

"Express yourself completely" means allowing our inner self to be the place from which we interact with the outer world. "Then keep quiet," because if you have expressed yourself completely, there is nothing more that needs to be said.

The lines "When it blows, there is only wind" and "When it rains, there is only rain" represent the pure characteristics of your personality.

"When the clouds pass, the sun shines through" is the key here. The clouds are the surface, and the sun is the essence. The clouds represent situations and circumstance; the sun is your indomitable nature.

We can fully express ourselves by cultivating the part of us that resides below the surface and is apportioned to everyone, regardless of background, culture, or station in life. This is our indomitable nature—an inner strength that increases in concentration and potency when put to work. It arrives in the challenges we face as we make our way through the uncertainties of life. It is a deep-seated characteristic that, when we're faced with dark and perilous situations that strip us of security, gives us the resolve to move on. It is a core attribute, an inner voice that cannot be ignored. That inner voice carries a message: Walk on. Never say die.

We can learn to be our authentic selves. We can train to respond to the difficulties of life. We can cultivate inner strength—the essential part of us, the sun that shines through.

You can develop inner strength without needlessly subjecting yourself to the endless trials and hardships that arouse this part of your being. You do so by developing faith. A faith in yourself: the act of letting go of preconceptions, and perceiving reality as the source that inspires a rise in your spirit. Each day is an opportunity to commit, prepare, and shape ourselves in this way through disciplined practice.

Every morning is a clean slate. We will experience a day of intention, circumstance, and perception unfolding in endless variations from daybreak until we lie down to sleep at night. The morning is an opportunity to begin creating a new version of yourself. It is scientifically true. The body expels dead cells and creates new ones every day. If each new cell contains the information of our bodies, then we want to make sure we are programming those cells with the best information possible. Our practice informs our bodies on a cellular level, and it encodes an intelligence that becomes more of our being over time. We strengthen ourselves by renewing ourselves at the cellular level.

This is one of the reasons why the T'ai Chi form we practice doesn't change: because the form is changing us! Over time and through repetition, our physique changes and our way of movement becomes more supple. These developments are visible to us, while below the surface we change on a cellular level. Our thinking becomes relaxed, lucid, and subconscious. Our entire organism is in a constant and subtle state of creating itself. The T'ai Chi form does not change—but you do.

T'ai Chi is a pathway to contemplation. When we play the form slowly, it is a meditation. In doing so, we move the ego to the side and free the subconscious mind to reveal our authentic self—the wellspring of inner strength. We are in a state of awareness without the cerebral, the thinking, the ego. This level of awareness illuminates our true nature, the essence of our individual humanity. In the East this is called *Te*.

Te, pronounced "day," means "by virtue of." It comes from our personal nature. If your action is contrived, or if there is any thought, agenda, goal, or expectation attached to it, then the action is not *Te*, because it is not rooted in your virtue.

The person working to satisfy a need, solve a problem, or lead an action is most impactful when they are being themselves. This person does not seek political leverage, more money, or reciprocal actions. Even if this person were to receive one or all these benefits—and even appreciate them—the benefits were not their motivation to act. They were simply a byproduct.

The person whose actions are from *Te* is indeed a wealthy person, because they act without expectation of reward. Any reward received will be in excess of their need. So, the unanticipated reward becomes part of their riches.

The word *virtue* has different shades of meaning. *Te* as virtue isn't defined as a strict moral standard. One meaning is "the capacity to act." For example, a village or town near a river has access to water for drinking, watering crops, and bathing. The river does not steer its path toward the town so that it can help; it simply flows as rivers do, and townspeople take what they need. But should the river surge and flood the crops or town, would this be considered an amorality? I think not. To surge and overflow, regardless of the damage it causes, is simply the nature of the river. And we accept that. But we have a hard time accepting that the same reality exists with another person's point of view, preference, allegiance, or reaction, assuming that it's a genuine response and not contrived as a scheme to control a situation.

Te can be summed up as doing without striving. You spontaneously respond to practical, social, professional, or political affairs with an unconscious command or power. You act unselfishly and your actions are natural and genuine because you don't seek gain.

Self-mastery free of self-awareness is power without force. In this context "without force" means not imposing or cutting against the grain. The key to mastering *Te* resides in *Wu-Wei*: not forcing.

When I heard the expression "rolling with the punches" as a child, it seemed to imply that I had to take the hit. And sometimes in life we do receive some real blows to the body, the mind, and our life. But the meaning of "rolling with the punches" began to change as I internalized the concepts of T'ai Chi Chuan.

Each technique in the T'ai Chi form originates from defense: meeting the attack, then neutralizing, redirecting, and issuing power. Through learning and practice I began to not fight against, but align with, the incoming force, regardless of its dimension and source. To achieve this, I needed inner strength. I had to have faith that the techniques are there for me. That meant that I had to let go of the ego. I had to trust my subconscious.

To have good T'ai Chi you must align with Tao, Te, and Wu-Wei. The T'ai Chi form is a physical representation of these principles. They are practiced daily like a mantra. Over the course of years of practice, these attributes trickle into your subconscious and integrate into your lifestyle. Like a sage or mystic, you recognize and know the principles, patterns, and tendencies occurring in nature and, by extension, among people. You interact from a natural source existing at a deeper level, beyond intellectual and emotional responses: you interact from your subconscious. This is the purest energy—your true power.

You also begin to truly understand that people's behavior, good or bad, is relative. For example, think of the course of history and how societal norms change. What was once unacceptable now may be considered respectable behavior. Elvis shaking his hips on television comes to mind. It caused an uproar back then but would hardly be noticed in the choreography of the modern pop star.

As leaders, lawmakers, managers, or parents, we have a better opportunity to make appropriate decisions if we understand how difficult it will be to impose strict laws or rules on the nature of others. It's better to understand their nature and then influence its direction, to not judge harshly when their actions don't align with our own view of the world. We may not like what someone did, but that doesn't necessarily mean they were wrong for doing it. If these are generally not dangerous people, then their tendencies are part of who they are.

I would rather have an imperfect but genuine person in my world than the overly righteous person who admits no fault, holds others to their own standards, imposes rules regardless of the level of relationship, and defends their personal view at any and all costs. This is not a person you can trust.

This person has a linear point of view and compartmentalizes things. They need predictability. When something unpredictable occurs, they attempt to control it. But it takes a lot of energy and force to impose such a will. It also leads to more disappointment. As this type of person ages and loses their strength and vitality, they become deeply bitter and insecure as nature's eternal patterns remain on course, appearing as chaos to them.

Why work so hard? Why not let life flow and align with it, approaching occurrences intelligently? Good or bad, the event won't last. Nothing does. But once you enter a situation that you might label as "bad," and all you seek is something "good," then you become stuck in the situation itself. It is now a fixed thing, like a photograph you're trapped in. This only creates more friction as the reality of life continues to move. Resist and you stay where you are, but allowing for your intuitive understanding will shed new light.

This is not meant to imply that we might experience life's vicissitudes in a purely detached and passive way. Feelings and emotions are part of our nature, too, and thus we must let them occur and pass. Suppress an emotion, and you're stuck again. Let the emotion occur and then move on. It is less stressful.

As the Tao states: *Express yourself completely; then keep quiet.*

* * *

Contrary to perceptions that the goal of T'ai Chi is to escape life, the solitude of practice and meditation is intended to master the self in order to function in the realities of the world. We must learn ourselves first, because nothing that has been created, organized, or built can measure up to the subtle complexity of you: a living organism. Every cell contains energy and information.

Our brain is more powerful and subtle than any computer. T'ai Chi is a medium to realize your virtue as the seed of inner strength. Practicing T'ai Chi deepens the connection and faith in these qualities and empowers you to correspond with the world on your own terms.

Attain knowledge, but then get out of your own way. Let go of strict doctrine, remove anxiety, and reside in awareness. Live your life. Respond as the situation requires.

The great Taoist scholars, priests, and sages understood that within self-knowledge was self-governance, which is above any written law. Their response was unapologetically consistent with their personal nature, regardless of circumstance. The lesson here is that external influence or circumstance, someone's opinion, or even an offensive or nasty comment does not need to be accepted as an absolute.

Some of these offenses are strategies intended to provoke a reaction—in many cases, anger, which is a loss of control. Loss of control is surrendering control to your opponent. Anger and loss of control is weakness, whereas calmness and composed behavior is inner strength. And you know what? That calm, cool demeanor is far more unsettling to the perpetrator than loss of temper, which they predict. You are unshakeable and indomitable. The T'ai Chi person responds to situations and moves on with their life.

When the clouds pass, the sun shines through.

Your authentic nature is revealed in these moments of true action. Because you haven't stopped to think about it. You simply responded. There was no consideration of acceptance, reputation, or status. There was no striving. There was only *Te*—your virtue. Our inner nature *is* our inner strength.

"But what if I make a wrong choice?" I can almost hear you say.

This choice you made has created a new condition and so now you respond again, and then again, until a natural and harmonic state returns. In times like these, which can be difficult, we learn the most about ourselves and our relationship to the world around us. The true teacher is experience.

Inspiration for Practice

PRACTICE AS YOU LIVE. Living the principles is the best way to express them in your T'ai Chi. There is no end. You will always discover a new depth of feeling. Through practice we purify these feelings so that we can understand ourselves more clearly. The path of T'ai Chi as introspection is a purification. It is in this transcendent experience that we discover our virtue and virtuosity.

Play your T'ai Chi form in the morning, imagining how your new healthy cells are alive in your being. Allow your virtue to emerge, like a glow from within. This will be more of a sense or feeling, so don't attempt to intellectu-alize, analyze, or label it. Just open the gate. Notice how you feel. Do you feel vibrant? More self-assured? Can you access this sensation again tomorrow or the day after through practice? Experiment and observe your feelings.

I LEARNED AN INNER
SECRET OF T'AI CHI

Why does T'ai Chi elicit a physical, mental, and—more than emotional, a *spiritual*—experience unlike anything else? For years I have practiced and observed how the subtle movements of the art were transforming me. Who or what I was at the beginning of my T'ai Chi session was different than at the end. What is it about T'ai Chi that stimulates such transcendence?

T'ai Chi ("grand ultimate"), or more specifically T'ai Chi Chuan ("grand ultimate fist"), is a martial art, and an effective one at that. To reach the level of effectiveness, you must experience its transcendence, which can only be revealed through your personal understanding, as informed by years of training and practice. The practice is a ritual that focuses on a pure motive, which is to achieve a pure mind. Having a pure mind enables you to experience each moment as it occurs without the interference of conscious thought.

Conscious thought is the tool we use for analysis, strategy, and projected outcomes. It is not a tool to be used when an instant response is required. Conscious thought occupies the mind with memories or future projections: images of what has occurred, or what *might* occur. It colors each experience with an opinion, like an ongoing commentary of the event's positive or negative impact on us. Some people are consciously thinking all the time. It boosts their confidence because they feel more alert. Being alert and being aware are different things, though.

Being alert is not to be confused with readiness. Being alert is being alarmed. Being alert and thinking on some level is important, but when you are occupied by conscious thoughts, you are inclined to anticipate based on past knowledge or an imagined future, not the existing reality. Conscious thought and anticipation do not ensure a correct response to the present moment. In a conflict, people often employ anticipation as a strategy when awareness is required. This erroneous approach causes anxiety and tension because it commits you to a direction, even though the cause or active event hasn't yet occurred. Once committed to a direction, you may have to withdraw, recoil, and reposition to address the actual attack, which inevitably came from another direction—the one that you did *not* anticipate. By then it is too late.

The mind has to play catch-up now, because conscious thought has created a lag in time. You are not in the flow of the event but instead are trying to process events that have already happened. In sparring that means you are constantly under attack and getting hit. Your true state of mind is revealed in these exchanges. Here is where

T'ai Chi's Pushing Hands and sparring drills expose a significant truth: that in the exchange you are essentially fighting two opponents, the other person and your own disordered thoughts.

Without a disciplined practice to quiet the mind, many people seek only to increase conscious thought, even when it's working against them. Consistent T'ai Chi practice moves away the cloud of conscious thought, enabling your mind to be more attentive. Awareness is a product of the unconscious—pure thought—because it sees things as they are, without the distraction of labeling and assigning opinions or values. It increases intelligence, and in doing so more fully empowers your interaction with people, events, and revelatory experiences.

T'ai Chi trains you to experience life in the present, just as it is. Preparing and practicing for readiness, and stilling the mind for unconscious mindful thinking (awareness), vitalizes your participation in life. The mind is clear and without expectation when functioning in its proper state. It exists in a middle ground that doesn't commit prematurely to a direction or intention. When an attack or conflict occurs, the mind simply responds. The unimpeded directness of the response is a result of pure thought.

Understanding this takes years of practice and contemplation. It slowly becomes more of a living truth. Over time, your perspective of conflict begins to change. So does your response.

Perhaps the most recognizable change is the realization that a verbal threat is not the same as an actual attack.

It seems obvious when you read it, but for someone experiencing a threat from an intimidating person, the threat seems real. But even when spoken from a large, intimidating person, the threat itself is just words, delivered with a level of emotional intensity. That doesn't mean you shouldn't take the threat seriously. You must. But you don't want it to trigger the fight or flight response unnecessarily or prematurely. That only escalates the encounter to the very thing you seek to avoid.

Remember, words alone are merely representations. Action is truth. A person threatening harm is very different from a person moving toward you with raised hands or a weapon. Maintaining a pure mind enables you to see the encounter and its level of threat more truthfully.

A strike in the form of a punch or kick can be regarded as a point of conflict. Do you focus on the strike? To focus on the strike is to focus on the sole source of pressure. This places the mind into a purely defensive mode. The mind begins to think about how to defend, which again creates a delay and cedes the advantage to the source of attack.

Instead, see the attack and realize that openings exist all around this single line of incoming force. The opening is where your opportunities are found. Sparring exemplifies this concept, but this truth exists in every level and form of conflict, including disagreements, competitive pressure at work or school, and social politics. When we focus only on the force of the attack and react, then we invariably react incorrectly and, most importantly, do not open our field of vision to all the opportunities that are available to us.

It's also important to recognize and remember that every action is imperfect. Unlike the conflicts you read about in books or watch in the movies, every clash has an element of chaos and unpredictability; every fight is raw and violent on some level. You will attack or defend in a certain way, but the reality is that your choice may not be effective every time. You are vulnerable to a counterstrike and may get hit. This is the reality of conflict—but you still must act.

Do you see how in this regard T'ai Chi is a representation of the act of living? T'ai Chi trains us how to respond to the incoming forces of life by flowing and finding opportunities. You are removing your patterns of struggle, which only frustrate you and deplete your energy in difficult situations. The key is simple: do not overthink. There's no perfect choice in life. This truth is epitomized in Robert Frost's classic poem "The Road Not Taken," which begins:

Two roads diverged in a yellow wood,
And sorry I could not travel both

Frost goes on to contemplate his choices and what future each path may hold:

Yet knowing how way leads to way, I doubted if I should ever
come back.

Think and choose, then move forward. The real flaw is remaining stuck at the fork in the road, caught in deliberation and seeking the perfect way. A T'ai Chi life is one of movement. Movement is where the intelligence of life is ever present.

T'ai Chi trains you to still the mind through meditation, complex techniques, and the labyrinth-like progression of the form. T'ai Chi Chuan is the next level of training. It maintains the stillness of meditation and forms while increasing the level of action and pressure. Over time you naturally begin to incorporate the stillness into the common actions of your life. The trials and contests from training and the challenges of daily living are key to your transformation as a human being.

Early training is focused on cultivating inner strength. This is a strength that is used to deal with events, obstructions, conflicts, setbacks, vulnerabilities, and disappointment, each of which carries a level of power over you. The distribution of that power changes when you have greater inner strength.

Next you discover your *power*: your capacity to act. T'ai Chi reveals that this power exists within you. The power of events will never subside or go away, but you can meet that power with your own, blending the two to shape your future, whatever it may be. Both powers belong to the grand power that exists in the universe, the grand ultimate: *T'ai Chi.* You have a greater sense of firmness in the realization that positive and negative forces coexist, and integrating them is your participation in the unending act of creation—the essence of life's eternal cycle.

Inspiration for Practice

EXPLORE. Use your practice time to explore a different way of moving, or a different rhythm, or a different emphasis. You don't need to adopt these explorations as a permanent way of doing things, but in exploring you discover what does or doesn't work. You'll naturally discover your own subtle form of expression. That is the art in martial arts.

TOMORROW
NEVER KNOWS

This work is meant to raise awareness. My experiences are not unique, but they are personal.

What I gleaned from observing and reflecting on these experiences, combined with direct and indirect instruction, reading, and practicing—and then breaking everything down and experimenting within the T'ai Chi art—were my answers. But my answers may not be yours. True development and transcendence take place within, not outside of you.

The way to develop your internal mode of experience is to gradually reduce outside interference. Over time you learn to listen to and live within life's law and realize that nothing in this world is more important. Coming to know the way of human nature through the study of life leads to self-understanding.

T'ai Chi is a discipline through which one discovers and then corrects and refines physical, mental, and emotion inadequacies. It teaches us to eliminate the waste that pollutes clear thinking while at the same time cultivating self-knowledge. This takes a lifetime to achieve.

There are those who wish to learn from external experience, or from image and appearance. But there are others who seek to find the secret meaning hidden within their encounters. Look deeply and be sensitive to your own feelings as well as the transformations in how you interact with the world. This is an awakening to life. To get to this place takes practice and a willingness to experience all that life will bring to you without judgment or remorse.

The T'ai Chi experience, much like a divine musical performance, reveals the inner flame of your power and potential. You must pursue an excellence that builds the self and yet is selfless. An excellence that empowers but includes responsibility. To allow yourself to be exposed, but with strength and compassion.

T'ai Chi is a beautiful display of art: physical refinement that can be used to hurt or heal. One learns to live beyond themselves and in doing so becomes more alive. The art is our physical link to an invisible world. Through practice we experience this hidden motivating force—a spirit, the essence of life itself. In the end, you must understand your own experience and knowledge and then synthesize it into a unique response to the events and encounters that make up your life. You must find a daily practice that builds and maintains that faith. Faith in yourself, and faith in the great mysterious source that exists beyond us.

You thrive in the world when you are aware of the continuity of change, that all things combine and reshape in endlessly repeating variations based on a few natural laws. Those events and challenges put questions to the soul, as Ralph Waldo Emerson has said, and the creation of our response will shape and reshape who we are. It forges our uniqueness. And it brings peace of mind. A peace of mind achieved not by avoiding the unpleasant, but by connecting with ourselves and our truth every day. Then we must live to that truth, our natural law, and make our statement in society not by protest or anger, but by living an independent life of continuity and variation. This is our life's evolution.

We can't control what happens in the world around us, but we can understand the silent flow of nature in each unfolding event. Instead of trying to control an outcome, we align with the source. We clear away the webs of confusion brought on by outside influence to discover a unique and textured life within our unique circumstance, without being lulled to an unconscious sleep by the illusion of a different or better life. T'ai Chi teaches us how to put excellence into every aspect of life. In doing so, we live in a constant act of creativity that makes for a full and more satisfying existence.

And tomorrow? Tomorrow is the unwritten reality. We may look to newscasters, pundits, and experts to provide their personal view of the future. For a short time, they may provide hope, or fear, but not the security that we seek. In the end we can only take a chance, living spontaneously and vulnerably.

A lifetime practice of T'ai Chi develops faith in ourselves to make a choice and then determine if that choice is harmonic or dissonant with our core truth. The consequence influences our next move. Because life is not lived in the temporary ups and downs, wins and losses, but in the movement itself. The pathway is chaotic. It is sloppy. It is risky. You may never feel prepared enough. The T'ai Chi way of life does not have a defined timetable for results. In the philosophy there are no clear good guys and bad guys, winners or losers. That is what keeps our life a mystery. T'ai Chi's hidden lessons teach a way to embrace this mystery as a lifelong expression in the art of living.

Appendix A:
T'AI CHI AND THE MUSICIAN

I was a musician long before I began training in martial arts. Once I started to train in T'ai Chi and kung fu, I noticed a change in my physical approach to music. Then a mental shift occurred. I sensed a connection between the two but couldn't describe what it was. Since then, I've spent my time as a practicing artist—music and martial— exploring how the two disciplines intersect. I believe that discovering a common element will mutually enhance the two, but more so, that I will uncover a hidden connecting root—a divinity—that harbors some sort of life force. It has been a fascinating journey.

I began practicing my T'ai Chi form to rhythm. Just like dancing, T'ai Chi in a rhythm enables me to physically feel that rhythm. Dancing tends to be quicker, so it can be hard to determine if you're exactly on the beat or not. And I'm not a dancer, anyway. I found that T'ai Chi was beneficial because I have enough time to observe for accuracy. Practicing T'ai Chi with a defined beat increases awareness of your body's movement through space over an interval of time. The slow tempo makes it more obvious when your movement arrives early or late.

T'ai Chi with rhythm allows you to relax into your body movement, which is one of the most significant benefits of this practice. Your posture improves, too. Your body becomes more settled, like water settles, which creates a fullness and sense of bottom to the notes you play on the instrument. You'll play with better intent, which improves the feeling of pulse and groove in the music. The quality of your expressed rhythm is increased.

T'ai Chi within a rhythm internalizes the feeling of your full physical movement in tempo, which translates to playing music with a stronger and more natural sense of time. This is different than a musician's common practice of focusing to improve rhythm only in the hands and feet. Drummers, for example, will become more aware of how their arms, hands, and sticks travel from one surface of a drum or cymbal across the open space to the next part of the instrument.

T'ai Chi can also benefit singers and horn or string players. These instruments seem to have fewer physical demands than drumming, but observe a virtuoso closely, and you'll see them fully engaged physically with their instrument. In his book *Themes and Variations*, renowned violinist and conductor Yehudi Menuhin describes the full use of his body, from the toes through the hips, up the vertebrae through the shoulders and wrist, to the fingertips touching his violin. That same kinetic sequence is encoded into every movement of T'ai Chi.

For the traveling musician, I can think of no better antidote to the physical stress of the travel/performance/travel cycle. You can do T'ai Chi anywhere at any time to rejuvenate or wind down after a long day. The enhanced performance and quality of life can make the difference between a good tour and a great tour.

Ultimately T'ai Chi is a practice that brings musicians in tune with themselves. I remember teaching T'ai Chi to a working musician. At our lesson I asked if she had been practicing what I gave her.

She shrugged and said, "Well, not really, no."

I then asked, "Have you ever walked on stage to perform without tuning up?"

She said no.

I said, "Then why do you start your day before getting yourself in tune?"

She made the change, and her daily life changed with it. And then so did the quality of her music because it now had more meaningful content and vibrantly communicated what it means to be alive. To me, this is the real purpose of music. Every instrument is a material extension of ourselves. It is a conduit that expresses our unconscious spirit emotionally through physical form—the body, our true instrument.

Appendix B:
T'AI CHI AND THE MOVIES

T'ai Chi has played a role in Chinese martial arts movies, albeit mostly as a supporting player. For instance, in an installment of the *Ip Man* movie franchise, *Ip Man 4*, Ip Man engages in an intense competition with a local T'ai Chi Sifu (instructor). I understand that this one sequence took twelve days to shoot.

T'ai Chi is occasionally the main feature in movies, such as *Tai Chi Master* (Jet Li), *Man of Tai Chi* (Keanu Reeves), *Tai Chi Zero*, and *Tai Chi Hero*. And although under the radar, T'ai Chi has made cameos in major Hollywood movies, where it's incorporated into scenes to express sophisticated fighting arts on a higher level. Some of the best-known examples include:

- Dalton (played by Patrick Swayze) training in the summer heat, shirtless, in the classic *Road House*. (I *know* that you have seen this movie. Everyone has.)

- Colin Farrell is drafted into a Special Ops unit in *The Recruit*. He's shown awkwardly training in

T'ai Chi as the recruits develop their skill in the dark arts.

- In the first *Lethal Weapon* movie, Sergeant Murtaugh (Danny Glover) says to Riggs (Mel Gibson): "They say you know martial arts and T'ai Chi."
- T'ai Chi takes a lighthearted turn when practiced by Robert DeNiro in *The Intern*.
- *The Killer Elite* stars James Caan as an elite mercenary and martial arts expert.

A cursory look on the internet surfaced the names of iconic celebrities who practice—or have practiced—T'ai Chi, including:

- Tom Brady, NFL quarterback
- RZA, member of the Wu-Tang Clan
- Mel Gibson, actor, producer, and director
- Adrian Paul, actor
- Terence Stamp, actor
- Lou Reed, rock musician
- Tony Visconti, rock producer (Lou Reed, David Bowie)
- Allen Ginsberg, Beat poet
- Iggy Pop, rock musician
- Bette Midler, singer and actress
- Marianne Faithfull, singer
- Gisele Bündchen, supermodel

And the list is growing. . . .

Appendix C:
T'AI CHI AND SPORTS

Remember the Titans is one of the all-time classic sports movies. It tells the story of a disparate team of high schoolers brought together by their coach to achieve a common goal. Through the experience each player discovers themselves, their humanity, and their greatness. It's a "must-see" sports movie.

One of the characters is Ronnie "Sunshine" Bass, who is admired by the high school girls. Not only is he handsome, but the girls are equally attracted to the exotic appeal of Sunshine's morning T'ai Chi workout. He puts those skills to work in a locker room fight, then later during the big game. T'ai Chi has a minor role in the movie, but it illustrates a major link between training in T'ai Chi and Western sports performance. And like the movie, T'ai Chi has been put to work by the NFL.

Steve Clarkson, a highly sought-after private coach known as the "quarterback guru," incorporates T'ai Chi into his training program for college and pro-level athletes. Clarkson worked with Tim Tebow when Tebow was with the New York Jets. Clarkson used T'ai Chi to improve Tebow's footwork and get his body aligned to work in concert with itself. Clarkson employed the same techniques for Terrelle Pryor during Pryor's time with the Oakland Raiders. The San Francisco 49ers employed George Chung, dubbed "the Bruce Lee of the NFL," for their training.

I became aware of this connection while teaching a group class. A young man began training, and I learned that he was a pitcher for his high school baseball team. I soon began to teach the Brush Knee technique. This has similarities to pitching, which includes establishing balance during the wind-up and leg lift, transferring weight from the back leg to the front, aligning the hips and shoulders, sinking and rotating the hips, and finally generating energy through the arm to release the ball. Practicing the principles of T'ai Chi improved this student's level of pitching over the course of the season.

Since then, I have worked with golf, volleyball, and hockey players seeking to increase their level of performance. They embraced the no-impact, no-stress, non-competitive element of T'ai Chi because it enabled them to improve their health, fitness, and body alignment, which enhanced their game without risk of injury. For injured players, T'ai Chi can be an excellent path to recovery.

The practice of T'ai Chi and its underlying Taoist principles offer benefits by helping direct the athlete's mind and body toward their higher potential, which is the essential goal of sports. Through T'ai Chi training, the athlete will come to understand their inner world. They will focus on excellence as the basis of self-worth, as opposed to a trophy, which is the visible reward.

T'ai Chi isn't on the radar of most sports trainers, but for those who know, it is recognized as excellent physical and mental training for competitive athletes. An athlete who patiently invests time to learn and master the subtle variations of an art like T'ai Chi can only improve personally and athletically. They can potentially emerge as a superior player of their game.

Appendix D:
RECOMMENDED READING

I am an eternal student and like to immerse myself in subjects I most enjoy. T'ai Chi is no different. Beyond learning the form and applications, I'm curious about the history and roots of the art. I like to learn why we practice the way we do, and what the benefits might be. In addition to the resources I've referenced throughout this book, this appendix provides a partial list of books I've found to be informative and inspirational. Each book listed here offers something slightly different, like viewing facets of a diamond. I encourage you to read these works and others that may enhance your T'ai Chi journey.

Aurelius, Marcus. *Meditations*. Mineola, NY: Dover Publications, 1997.

Chow, David, and Richard Spangler. *Kung Fu History, Philosophy and Technique*. Burbank, CA: Unique Publications, 1982.

Chuen, Master Lam Kam. *The Way of Energy: Mastering the Art of Internal Strength with Chi Kung Exercise.* New York: Simon & Schuster, 1991.

Emerson, Ralph Waldo. *Self-Reliance.* Mineola, NY: Dover Publications, 2016.

Hodge, Stephen. *Tao Te Ching.* London: Godsfield Press, 2002.

Huang, Chungliang Al. *Embrace Tiger, Return to Mountain: The Essence of Tai Ji.* Philadelphia: Singing Dragon, 1973.

Mitchell, Stephen. *Tao Te Ching.* New York: Harper & Row, 1988. *

Rosenfeld, Arthur. *Tai Chi: The Perfect Exercise, Finding Health, Happiness, Balance and Strength.* Cambridge, MA: Da Capo Press, 2013.

Tzu, Lao. *The Dao De Jing: A Qigong Interpretation.* Translated by Dr. Jwing-Ming Yang. Wolfeboro, NH: YMAA, 2018.

Watts, Alan, with Al Chung-liang Huang. *Tao: The Watercourse Way.* New York: Pantheon Books, 1975.

Wayne, Peter M., and Mark L. Fuerst. *The Harvard Medical School Guide to Tai Chi.* Boulder, CO: Shambhala, 2013.

Wei, Lindsey. *The Valley Spirit: A Female Story of Daoist Cultivation.* Philadelphia: Singing Dragon, 2013.

Wile, Douglas. *T'ai-Chi Touchstones: Yang Family Secret Transmissions.* Brooklyn, NY: Sweet Ch'i Press, 1983.

---

* This is the first version I read. I have used Mitchell's interpretation throughout this book.

Wollering, Loretta M. *Anatomy of Fitness: Tai Chi: The Trainer's Inside Guide to Your Workout.* Melbourne, Australia: Hinkler Books, 2016.

Yang, Dr. Jwing-Ming. *The Root of Chinese Qigong, Secrets for Health, Longevity & Enlightenment.* Wolfeboro, NH: YMAA Publications, 1989.

Yang, Dr. Jwing-Ming. *Taijiquan, Classical Yang Style.* Wolfeboro, NH: YMAA Publications, 1999.

Zhuang, Henry. *The Mind Inside Tai Chi: Sustaining a Joyful Heart.* Wolfeboro, NH: YMAA, 2015.

INDEX

ACKNOWLEDGMENTS

Billie Fitzpatrick, you guided with a steady hand, and your questions and critique were always wrapped in encouragement. Thanks for helping me make the abstract more clear.

Boris Gluzberg, beyond a colleague, you are a friend in every regard. Thank you for thinking beyond the norm and then knowing who to speak to about it.

Darlene Famiglietti, I could bounce any idea, inspiration, or notion off you for reflection and meaning. Your thoughtfulness and enthusiasm energized me through this work.

Cathy Calame, your questioning eye and enthusiastic commentary were much needed and much appreciated at this point in the book.

Greg Brower, we wrote our books in parallel, which kept me motivated and moving. That, plus a pint and discussions on philosophy, politics, religion, and music. Who could ask for more? Now it is your turn.

Mark Schnurman, an old friend came full circle for a more fulfilling friendship. I learned as much from our sessions as you, and am forever grateful for the gentle nudge: "So, how is the book coming along?"

Violet Li, your passion and commitment have been an inspiration. Your knowledge of the art and technical expertise are vital. Thank you for your suggestions on some of the finer points. I am pleased to call you a friend and colleague.

Sifu Gus Kaparos, you had the *audacity* to teach this late bloomer more than a technique, form, or self-defense. What I was learning was a self-discipline that cultivates the power each of us has within: mental, physical, and spiritual. The true art is the transcendence of the self.

Shannon Donnelly, intelligence and clarity, inner strength and passion, vision and conviction. A beautiful combination. I wish I were that together at your age. It is my hope that the completion of this work shows you that anything is possible. And that *You*, my dear, can do anything you want. You showed me that many times while I tried to figure out how to make this little book idea fly.

Jeanne Donnelly, for better or worse, you wound up with a dreamer. Thank you for always listening without questioning and for all the days and nights you were a widow in effigy while I chased inspiration. I am sure it has not always been easy. But hopefully not boring, either.

ABOUT THE AUTHOR

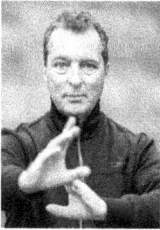

Bill Donnelly has made an art of his life. He is a musician and composer, author, martial artist, entrepreneur, career expert, and teacher. Bill has been practicing T'ai Chi Chuan for over twenty-five years. He teaches the philosophical, health, and martial elements of the art, which he studied and developed in addition to kung fu with Sifu Kaparos of the Green Cloud Martial Arts Academy in New York.

Bill has been invited to present workshops and speaking engagements around the New York area and is a frequent demonstrator at World T'ai Chi Day events. He continues to teach T'ai Chi's traditional applications, as applied to conflict resolution, life, and business strategies, in group or private sessions for corporations, executives, entrepreneurs, and individuals.

For private instruction, appearances, or speaking engagements, visit *www.privatetaichi.net.*

www.ingramcontent.com/pod-product-compliance
Lightning Source LLC
Chambersburg PA
CBHW052017030426
42335CB00026B/3175